REFLEXOGNOSY

A Shift in Paradigm

Gateway to Health Through the Feet

By Christine Issel and Sandra B. Rogers

New Frontier Publishing
P.O. Box 246654
Sacramento California 95824 USA
PH/FAX: 916-455-5381
E-mail quantum@ns.net
www.ns.net/~quantum/

Cover design by Lena Hugi

ISBN: 0-9625448-9-2

First Printing: April 2000

10 9 8 7 6 5 4 3 2 1

The information in this book is not intended as a substitute for medical care. If you have a health problem, consult a medical professional.

This book is available at a special discount when ordered in bulk quantities. Contact the publisher for details.

To the inquiring mind and those students who dare to be different by taking Reflexognosy on as a clinical discipline.

REFLEXOGNOSY™

Gateway to Health Through the Feet

TABLE OF CONTENTS

ACKNOWLEDGMENTS

Texts such as this only occur because many people have contributed either directly or indirectly. Some are not aware of their influence and others have worked tirelessly to bring this book into reality. To Ronny, my life partner, who works endlessly behind the scenes ensuring that my life runs smoothly and is always there allowing me the freedom and flexibility I need to chase my dreams I am grateful. Marge and Mandy, my friends and staff who are able to determine what it is I really mean when I think in shorthand, have been a blessing. They have also provided me the space to 'get on with it.' Richard Kobylarz, a Melbourne podiatrist, who assisted me in developing my clinical experience, has provided valuable assistance with the development of Reflexognosy. My lecturing team who has remained enthusiastic over many years as the paradigm has shifted and provided much needed support. All my students have been my teachers. Each student has assisted me in this journey. They have all played a major role and will continue to do so. A special note of thanks to two students: Mary Gibson of Canada and Gretchen Schaff of the United States. Both have been outstanding in their support of the work.

We are also indebted to Lorena Pollard of Los Angeles and Pamm Brittain of Melbourne for their editing and proofreading skills; to Alonzo Bartley of Toronto for his review and technical assistance with the scientific portion of this work; and to Billie J. Scott, Patricia Bowman and Joesph Horan for their invaluable aid in the production process. And of course, to our clients who have allowed us the privilege to work with them and their health issues using this much loved discipline, we are deeply grateful. Without them we would not be able to validate our hypotheses.

S.R. & C.I.

FOREWORDS

The only limits are, as always, those of vision
—James Broughton

No major advancement takes place without vision. Visionaries are also pioneers. Pioneering means to dare to think differently. Pioneering means to have courage. Visionaries see beyond the prevailing model, or thought forms upon which most of the world bases a decision at a given time, and challenge the very foundation of the establishment. Pioneers see the necessity of change to a model. At first, pioneers are ridiculed. Then they and their ideas are tolerated. Finally many years later the ideas put forth by pioneers are accepted by their profession and eventually by the public. As reflexologists, until we change the model of our present thinking and bring our education up to recognized standards we will not advance into the professional ranks which we deserve.

Today, we are called upon to be pioneers, to expand our thinking in new directions and depths. Much of the information contained within this work is already known or perceived in various professions, but it is seen here from a new angle requiring a slight shift in thought.

Thank goodness there are pioneering and inquiring minds in the world that make us question and examine our model. The most dynamic, creative and questioning mind I know is Sandi's. She has acted as a catalyst by continually pushing the frontiers of my knowledge as well as those of her other students. She is constantly asking why, when most of us just take things blindly at face value. One thing we both have always agreed on is that working on the feet is the most powerful healing modality there is because of the profound influence the feet have on health. I am also thankful for Sandi's patience in this project and her trust in letting me put words in her mouth. The writing of this book has taken longer than either one of us ever envisioned in the beginning.

This work asks the reader *to think*, not necessarily to agree. It encourages you to dare to be a pioneer and a visionary, to bring a new level of understanding to your work with the feet, and to re-evaluate the role of feet in health.

Christine Issel
Sacramento, California USA
April 2000

Heaven is under our feet as well as over our heads.
—Henry David Thoreau

When I initially thought about a book on Reflexognosy™[1] I was very much uncertain about how to go about it. The publication of this text has been one of my greatest learning experiences, and continues to be so. This work is literally an extension of thinking and collaborating with such a probing mind as Christine's. I thank Christine for having the courage to participate in this project. Not only has she worked beyond all expectations to bring the text into reality, she is a wonderful friend in the truest sense of the word as she provides creative balance for me. Over the years our relationship has been very rewarding.

Today basic values in all areas of our lives are changing at an alarming rate. This is especially true in health care. The population at large is looking for answers to their many health problems and reflexognosy will be of enormous assistance in this quest. However, if reflexognosy is to achieve its full stature in the service of humanity, it must, like most other developing fields before it, base its philosophy upon science, both social and anthropological. The way of developing this foundation is through education and training of practitioners to the highest level possible.

There is a wealth of knowledge throughout the world that bears relevance to the educational needs of those who work with the feet. It is now time that **all** the literature from different thoughts, concepts, and perceptions be pooled to strengthen the foundation of our knowledge. To this aim our book is dedicated. This work is designed to contribute to the foundations from which we work by first challenging and discussing present hypotheses. This in turn, offers an opportunity for a shift in paradigm by asking the reader to question and think. Reflexognosy is a blend of many thoughts brought together for the first time. Readers are called upon to develop and use critical thinking as a tool to assist understanding and professional development. This book will pose many questions. It will challenge the focus of all complementary health practitioners and provide an educational tool for the advancement of the field. Many may feel some concepts are unsettling and lead to confusion, but keep in mind that confusion or chaos is the first step to growth and clarity.

---

[1] Reflexognosy is defined as the application of appropriate pressure to the legs and feet by the hands of a trained practitioner to bring about physiological and psychological changes stimulating subtle energies. Refer to Chapter 3 for more information.

As the understanding of feet and the role they play in health grows and gains credibility, the field must maintain a wholistic balance between its art and science—our heart, head, and hands. Previous education has been on skill development, our hands-on techniques. Now we must focus on feeding our minds and understanding our hearts in order to blend art and science in a balanced order.

It should be noted, that I too, began by working within reflexology and the concept of reflexes. In order to understand the process I wrote about it in *Professional Reflexology for Everyone*. However, I then evaluated each and every concept. I questioned the mechanism by which amazing results were achieved. At first, I too was blinded by results—the application and the outcomes. The result of my searching has led to many questions being answered, and to this combined text. Through this latest work I am confident that students and other health care professionals will gain a deeper understanding of this valuable healing science known as Reflexognosy which works with the foot and leg. This is not the final work, only the beginning. The true challenge is to keep questioning and make improvement so that the beneficiaries, our clients, will be exposed to a great therapy with the practitioner having a full understanding of their discipline.

This discipline is in its infancy. The unique individuals who come to practice Reflexognosy in the future will play a major role in shaping the destiny of this work. Those who graduate and apply the therapy will be taking the first steps in research. Their observations and results will be monitored via the Global Reflexognosy Research Institute for Professionals (G.R.R.I.P.) in Melbourne. G.R.R.I.P. is a not for profit research foundation who will analyze the results and put them forth for academic and scientific review.

We are all like-minded, in that, each of us wants to contribute to society in some way. Today health care is entering an era of dynamic change. Reflexognosy can be a major contributor to new health care programs in the world community. It does not require costly equipment, it is inexpensive to apply, and fully portable.

To all future students, welcome to a very exciting field of health care. To everyone: never stop questioning and learning.

Find happiness in every moment,
Sandi Rogers
Melbourne, Victoria Australia
April 2000

Chapter 1

The Journey

A journey of a thousand miles starts with the first step.
—Chinese Proverb

In 1938 when Eunice Ingham published *Stories the Feet Can Tell* she called for readers to contribute to her efforts to validate reflexology: "So let me say should anyone, physician or layman, after a careful study and application of this method, have any valuable suggestions in the form of an explanation to offer, I will be glad to hear from them. Like every new development, it must prove its efficiency to many a doubting skeptic, *before being accepted as an established fact.*"[1] [emphasis added by Rogers & Issel]

Years later Ingham again poses the same request in *Stories the Feet Have Told* (1951). "I would like to see more research work done on this subject [reflexology] and would be glad to hear from anyone as to new developments in this field."[2]

In these statements Ingham was asking readers to apply critical thinking to the observations and theories she sets forth. She also wanted these ideas tested through the hands-on application of practical skills. All this was for the develop-

ment and advancement of reflexology. Unfortunately over the years people have accepted what she wrote as fact and not questioned the premise upon which she based her work. As a result, a review of reflexology literature indicates that the theories behind the current paradigm do not hold up to academic scrutiny. This is not to deny the effectiveness of the application of pressure to the feet. It is probably the most potent and cost effective healing discipline there is, and it has the distinction of being non-invasive. However, the point remains, practitioners of today owe it to their field to investigate the results they obtain.

Ingham (1951) also cautions her readers, "Those who have been studying human history will acknowledge that man has not learned all there is to know on any given subject and probably never will. Knowledge, like time and space, seems to be infinity [infinite], and to feel that the saturation point has been reached is a grave danger."[3]

Undoubtedly, the fear of

change and the fear of being challenged, keeps us clinging to our familiar standards and our old belief systems. A feeling of loyalty to our teachers may also prevent us from expanding our educational horizons. But we need to listen to our intuition when it keeps nudging us to explore other avenues and thoughts, in short, *to think*. We owe it to ourselves and to our chosen work to examine our subject from all angles. None of us owns our discipline; we are merely custodians of its future. We must cherish the role that we play and leave a profession as our legacy. This can only be accomplished by questioning the theories of our past and applying critical thinking in searching for answers. From this platform a discipline grows or is surpassed for more credible theories.

Education is a life-long adventure of pushing the frontiers of our knowledge. It is a process, and is not a matter of accumulating facts or information and regurgitating them. The educational process requires the use of critical thinking. It is essential to question what we are learning, not simply accept it on blind faith. Believe it or not, just because something is in print or espoused by some 'authority' does not make it true. It is the truth from their perspective. It is the student's responsibility therefore to question, reflect, and apply discernment. It is in this way that education leads to advances in knowledge. Every questioning student becomes the teacher for their teacher, and the cycle continues.

Critical Thinking

Jane Scott and Ronald Markert in their article on the relationship between critical thinking and success in medical school quote an earlier definition of critical thinking by Ennis (1962) as the narrow concept of "correctly assessing statements." Today, this definition has been broadened to include problem solving based on "intellectual curiosity, active learning, attitudes, knowledge, and reasoning skills."[4] Scott and Markert (1994) in a study involving medical students reached the conclusion that critical thinking can be an indication of academic success specifically during the pre-clinical years of a medical education. Brookfield (1987) offers relevant information to students when he writes: "Learning to think critically is one of the most significant activities of adult life. When we become critical thinkers we develop an awareness of the assumptions under which we, and others, think and act. We learn to pay attention to the context in which our actions and ideas are generated. We become skeptical of quick-fix solutions, of single answers to problems, and of claims to universal truth. We also become open to alternative ways of looking at, and behaving in the world."[5]

Students heeding this advice attempt to conceptualize information and search out possible reasons as part of the process in their education.

Critical thinking is not just an intellectual exercise which involves the logical left hemisphere of the brain. Feelings, intuitions, sensing, and emotional responses—activities of the right hemisphere of the brain which is more intuitive and creative—are all part of this wholistic process. Reasoning and drawing your own inferences is a process and not an outcome. It is reflecting with discernment. The lecturer's responsibility is to ensure that this occurs. In this way critical thinking can be a productive and positive process. For within the process is an inherent respect, appreciation of creativity and innovations, diversity of values and behaviors, all of which bring about a sense of our own humility through an awareness that the ideas and thoughts of others can be just as correct as our own. Rather than meaning to find fault, in its strictest sense, critical thinking implies an attempt at objective analysis so as to determine both the merits and faults before forming a judgment. In their study, Scott and Markert (1994) found that, in order to be the most successful, "Students need to evaluate relationships between words and statements and the use of absolute, qualifying, and conditional terms. Students must also evaluate whether the background statement supports the decision."[6] This formula helps the individual distinguish lies from truth and fact from fiction.

Those in wholistic disciplines can ill afford not to be critical thinkers. Their growing professions are in need of answers to complex challenges that threaten their credibility in this world of science and their viability in the market place. In some foot work disciplines, claims have been made regarding the feet that produce a threat to their very existence if scrutinized closely. Statements are based on wishful thinking and hypotheses that are unable to be validated with research. Deductions have been drawn from information that is not consistent with anatomy and physiology. Evaluations have been based on application and outcomes

and their interpretation not critically assessed.

Can we not answer Ingham's challenge without appearing to be disrespectful? Most scholarly arguments in relation to the feet stem from emotions and not fact. Theories are offered with little or no interest in the science and theory behind what is claimed and taught. The basis of this educational model is mechanically oriented. Instructional time is spent on learning charts and techniques of how to 'fix' the client's symptoms with little thought to the body-mind-spirit connection.

Tactile practitioners have great concern for those with whom they work. Yet, in some groups educational short cuts are taken by setting up a system that moves more and more toward procedures, tools, and a limited number of standard techniques. Questions about values, concerns, spirituality, love, caring, and meaning in illness and care giving, all have taken a back seat to the illusion of objectivity and 'skills based outcomes'.

People tend to stay in the 'comfort zone' of their dominant brain hemisphere and process every situation according to either a right or left brain preference. In tactile disciplines the dominance appears to be right brained due to the very nature of the art, and the fact that most practitioners are right brained orientated. For many, asking questions in an inquiring way about previously accepted ideas is anxiety producing and may seem too left brained. They may feel fearful of the consequences that might arise from teachers and peers when questioning long held dogmas and sacred cows. However, only in braving possible resentment

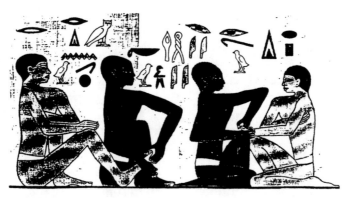

Work on the hand and foot 5,000 years ago in Ancient Egypt.

and attack can progress be made in understanding a therapy. The ultimate beneficiaries of this exercise will be the clients.

An example illustrating blind acceptance, without the application of critical thinking or academic rigor, is the belief that an Egyptian pictograph is proof of the existence of the practice of reflexology in Egypt five thousand years ago. Looking at the evidence, first one must put things in perspective and remember that the pictographs in the tomb are extensive and depict hundreds of illustrations that should be read in *combination*, not deciphered in isolation. Second, the pictographs taken together, as a single unit, represent life at the time—or perhaps in this case various physical procedures for the different stages of life from birth to death.

It can be agreed that the pictograph indicates a physical procedure, but in what context? An academic review of reference material from the Old Kingdom does not support the notion of the application of reflexology. Ghalioungui (1965), an Egyptian writing about his culture, refers to the pictograph as the demonstration of massage. Badawy (1976), another respected authority on the tomb, notes on the other hand,

that the pictograph, "representing the treatment of hands and feet, sometimes called manicure and pedicure." But he himself describes the scene as representing minor surgery. He justifies his position by writing, "as a result of walking barefoot, minor accidents and ailments requiring surgery must certainly have been common."[7]

In the *Illustrated History of Surgery* by Haeger (1988) Egyptian medicine is described as a "peculiar blend of superstition, ceremony and rational thinking."[8] If a patient's complaint was thought to have a tangible and natural cause, the patient went to the doctor; if the cause appeared more complicated or mysterious, a priest was consulted.

An objective review of the pictograph would indicate the belief in the value of touch as a diagnostic tool. According to a text cited by Haeger, the French scholar and Egyptian translator, Labat, felt the pictograph could indicate assessment of the body for tuberculosis. Tuberculosis was rampant at the time. Cold hands and warm feet are a classic sign of tuberculosis. This is accompanied by sweating and disturbed heart activity. Is it possible all these indicators were being examined in the pictograph? These same diagnostic procedures are used in determining tuberculosis today and they have nothing to do with reflexology.

Another hypothesis when viewing the pictographs of the tomb together as a single unit representing life at the time, is that the practitioners are assessing the pressure needed to deaden the pain as a pre-surgical procedure. It appears the pictograph could illustrate some kind of preparation for surgery because the other pictographs in the tomb show other surgeries like the practice of dentistry, circumcision, etc. Pressure applied to points may have produced a calming effect prior to surgery or childbirth. As a prelude to surgery, the hieroglyphic as translated by The Papyrus Institute in Cairo, "Do not hurt me" and the reply, "I shall act so you praise me" makes more sense.

Whatever the explanation, the assumption that it is reflexology demonstrates a lack of critical thinking skills and cannot be substantiated without further study. Critical thinking is a never-ending spiral of inquiry with four initial steps:

1. Identifying and challenging assumptions that underlie our beliefs.

2. Reflect, with skepticism, on supposedly fixed beliefs. Just because an idea is accepted by everyone does not mean that we have to believe in its innate truth without first questioning it, or working with it to see if it is a truth from our perspective.

3. Exploring and imagining alternatives. Subsequently those alternatives must be tested by research to either prove or disprove our

view. Whether that is literary, historical, social or scientific research, all must be conducted with an open mind toward what may be uncovered along the way.

4. Once again reflect on what has been uncovered and begin the process all over again.

Through the development of critical thinking we grow personally, professionally and culturally. We, as human beings, are not static and mechanistic. Nor, one would hope, is a profession. Therefore, old theories need to be questioned and our minds open to new concepts.

A close friend, Gretchen Schaff, from Philadelphia, has a crutch in her kitchen that dates from the American Civil War of the 1860s. It is a wooden apparatus and rather crude in design. It usually just leans against the wall with no one taking notice of it.

One morning over breakfast we were discussing the need for professions to grow and develop. We were noting that some people have a resistance to change, espousing there is no need to change and stand on the fact that they get results. "Why question or change, let's just stay with the status quo," they say.

Looking at the crutch, Gretchen likened professions to the crutch. She said, "You know, this crutch offers very good advice. Imagine what it would be like for people who need to use a crutch if in the past there were no questions posed as to how things could be better? How the crutch could be improved for the comfort of the injured? Who could offer such advice? The range of professions is extensive:

from the designer to the craftsmen who manufacture the device, to the physician who assesses the restrictions in the physiology through usage, to the hands-on practitioners who assess the physiological reactions. The list goes on."

If no one used critical thinking, the first crutch, the crude, wooden heavy apparatus would never have improved. True, the lame could still shuffle along, but circulation to their arms would be adversely affected due to poor mechanics, etc. The improvements we see in the equipment to aid the injured are truly amazing. This is due to the fact that professionals kept posing questions and assessing how things could be improved, never accepting the initial results. The mechanisms by which results could be improved were assessed and analyzed. To this present day these questions are still being posed in regard to the design of medical equipment like the crutch.

So too, will reflexognosy continue to question, as we do not want to be likened to the crutch from the Civil War, but as a modern device whose initial design has been improved and continues to evolve.

In some tactile disciplines authors and teachers around the world over many years have not reflected and examined statements by their predecessors. Instead they have restated information and presented theory as fact without demanding supporting evidence. Students have not been invited to question. This is not to criticize history or our predecessors, for the ideas put forth by writers and researchers must be reviewed in the framework of their time, and not with today's knowledge. But we must build on the past

and expand into the future utilizing past observations and information for the benefit of our community.

Good science is asking good questions. To serve in the best interest of our clients critical thinking is called for. We must look at what we are doing, build on the knowledge we have, trust our intuition, and ask, why?

To ask, "Why are things the way they are?" and "How might things be different?" does not necessarily entail the destruction of the ideas, or values under analysis. We must never cease to ask 'why' because failure to develop critical thinking, fails to free us from habitual ways of thinking and perceiving, and it also fails to develop a profession. Old myths and incorrect assumptions in the light of today's scientific knowledge will continue to be propagated to the detriment of a discipline. Teachers have the prime responsibility for developing critical thinking skills in themselves and their students, of encouraging its use by acting as catalysts for discussion and inquiry, by welcoming questions, fostering creativity, and displaying an openness to a diversity of interpretations of any particular topic or theory while withholding criticism and disagreement with the student who is expressing critical thinking skills. This is no easy task, but to do otherwise is to favor dogma and the status quo over evolving knowledge.

As Brookfield (1987) concludes, "Taking the risk to think critically, and to realize in our actions the insights we gain through this, is one of the most powerful activities of adult life.... We see the future as open to our influence. We regard the world as changeable through our own individual actions and through collective action in concert with others.... We do not accept the idea that because things are the way they are now, they must always be this way. And we do not think that we (or anyone else) have the ultimate answer to life's ambiguities and problems. But we do have confidence in knowing that those things in which we believe, and the actions we take arising out of these beliefs, spring from a process of careful analysis and testing against reality—in other words from critical thinking."[9]

As important as critical thinking appears to be, it is rarely taught at any educational level. Too often critical thinking is thought of as an academic exercise with no practical application in life. However, as Brookfield stated, it is a process we can apply to everyday challenges throughout life. Therefore, as students of the world, by applying this concept we will be serving our selected vocation, clients and ourselves as participants of life. The future growth of any profession, depends on the joint cooperative use and respect for critical thinking. It is in the spirit of critical thinking and the adventure of education that this book is written. It is hoped it will expand your thinking, start you questioning long held beliefs, and query what is found within these pages.

As Erich Fromm (1950) states, "...man's ability to search for truth is held to be inseparably linked to the attainment of freedom and independence."[10] Our ability to develop and use critical thinking skills may very well prove to be the one thing that will preserve and advance the profession as a separate field of study and work, while it may also be used

to complement many other disciplines.

Should you choose to continue reading this work you will be embarking on a journey that will challenge your belief systems. Hopefully it will prove to be enjoyable and enlightening. It will lead to an awareness of just how important attention to the feet and legs is in the healing process. We must go beyond the technical aspects of the work. We must delve deeply into the philosophical basis of the work with an open-mind to improve our understanding of the reality of nature. We must be wholistic in our theoretical approach through the examination of the many different health practices that involve working with the feet, and glean the information that is relevant to us. In this way we will begin to understand in real terms why such profound results are achieved via the feet and legs. In turn we will also be able to express the importance of our work in true professional wholistic terms to other health care professionals and our clients.

Are other tactile disciplines working on the feet, asking the wrong questions? Are they locked into Newtonian physics concepts? Is 18th-19th century science being used to explain a 21st century phenomena?

In her book Ingham (1951) used the most current analogy of her time and likened the nerves of the body to an electrical system. "The nerves of our body may be likened to an electrical system. It will be our ability to make the normal contact with the electricity in the ground, through our feet and from the elements or atmosphere surrounding us, that will determine the degree of power we are able to manifest in the

7

proper functioning of these glands." She continues, "Trying to get a normal contact when there is congestion in these nerve terminals in the feet is like trying to put a plug into a defective fixture."[11]

That was fifty years ago. However, thirty years later scientific thought and work expanded to the point where it was felt the body worked chemically with the release of hormones and other substances. Then ten years ago with further discoveries it was believed the body worked electromagnetically through dimensions of subtle energies and in this way to realms beyond the physical. Science does advance in its theories as new evidence comes to light and so should all disciplines.

To never ask questions or try to explain results borders on negligence and limits progress. The beneficiaries of questioning are both the public and the profession. This book is guaranteed to make you think and question. It is designed to take up Eunice Ingham's challenge to find the answers to the questions she posed in her books. Instead of accepting her thoughts as fact, this treatise is an attempt to apply critical thinking and current scientific knowledge to her theories and those of others. It hopes to bring about a shift in paradigm to the concepts held by tactile practitioners. The journey is based on anatomy and physiology of the foot and leg and quantum physics' concepts of the oneness and inter-relatedness of everything in the universe as applied to the body. Our aim is to work with the 'being' of our client and provide a discipline for those who wish to work with people and not conditions.

There is one very fortunate circumstance common to all systems of healing. That is that the human body is a wonderful creation which often recovers in spite of treatment and not because of it. However, it is the contention of the authors that the feet do offer the most valuable "Gateway to Health and Healing" through the hands of experienced and properly trained reflexognosists. Reflexognosy is the most complementary therapy in the healthcare field.

In any case whether you wish to pursue the practice of working with the feet as a professional practitioner or as a client, it is hoped after reading this text, you will never look at the feet and legs in quite the same way again.

---

[1] Ingham, Eunice. *Stories the Feet Can Tell*, Ingham Publishing, St. Petersburg, Florida, USA, 1938, pg. Introduction.

[2] Ingham, Eunice. *Stories the Feet Have Told*, Ingham Publishing, St. Petersburg, Florida, USA, 1951, pg. 32.

[3] Ibid. pg. 23.

[4] Scott, Jane and Ronald Markert. "Relationship Between Critical Thinking Skills and Success in Preclinical Courses". *Academic Medicine* V.69, November 1994, Pg. 20-24.

[5] Brookfield, Stephen D. Developing *Critical Thinkers*, Jossey-Bass Publishers, San Francisco, 1987, pg. ix.

[6] Scott, Jane and Ronald Markert, Pg. 20-24.

[7] Badawy, Alexander. *The Tomb of Nyhetep-Ptah at Giza and the Tomb of 'Ankhm'ahor at Saqqara*, University of California Press, Berkeley, 1978, pg. 19.

[8] Haeger, Knut. *Illustrated History of Surgery*, Bell Publication, New York, 1988, pg. 24.

[9] Brookfield, pg. 254.

[10] Fromm, Erich. *Psychoanalysis and Religion*, New York, Bantam Books, 1950, pg. 76.

[11] Ingham, Eunice. (1951), pg. 10.

Chapter 2

Defining the Theoretical Base of Foot Work

In therapy, first do no harm.
Life is short, art is long, the occasion is fleeting,
experience deceitful and judgment difficult.
—Hippocrates

Work on the feet can include such professions as orthopedics, podiatry, chiropractics, physical therapy, massage and other body work. Reflexology is also a popular form of foot work. Chart 1 on page 10 is a literature review of this therapy. The statements were taken from a group of reflexologists during a class. Their search of the literature confirms that the commonly held beliefs in print lead to confusion and a lack of stability in the curriculum. The comments are *their* opinions of what they found in the literature. They are used here to provide an exercise in critical thinking and to clearly demonstrate from where our interests have developed. The questions posed lead us on our own journey of discovery.

These are just some of the claims made by authors about how reflexology works or what it does. Authors of these statements offer no scientific validation of their hypotheses. Claims are often accompanied by anecdotal and empirical information as proof of the validity of statements. Each writer, in essence, asks the reader to accept their claims 'because they say so.'

However, the scientific model, or method of observation, is not concerned with our tactile skills, or how it *feels*, or how our clients *like* it. This model wants to know simply does it or does it not work, and if it works, what are some of the anatomical and physiological mechanisms by and through which it works. It wants to know how we can effectively bring about changes to the rest of the body using the medical model based on the tissue that is housed in the feet and the traditional principles of anatomy and physiology. It wants to know what research has been conducted to validate our claims. Therefore, as an exercise, let us *unemotionally* and *objectively* play devil's advocate by questioning the

The Theoretical Reasons for the Responses Obtained in Foot Work Based on Literature Review	
• Electro-Chemical response	• Works through the nerve endings
• Promotes endorphin release	• Works like acupuncture
• Proprioception	• Promotes relaxation and rest
• Unconscious response of the nervous system	• Promotes lymphatic drainage
• Locomotion/walking	• Improves circulation
• Communication between the zones	• Revitalizes energies
• Connective Tissue Massage	• It is a science and an art
• Energy systems/pathways	• Good preventative health care
• Stimulates creativity and productivity	• Works through zones
• Balances the chi energy	• Mirrors the body
• Weak muscles in the feet cause pressure	• Reduces Pain
• Autonomic nerve reflex response stimulating internal organs, muscles and glands	• Works through a reflex action
	• Pressure on any part of a zone effects all organs lying in that zone
• Different systems of the body are effected and cleansed	• Dissolves crystal deposits
• Is the same as a foot massage	• Is a diagnostic tool
• Revitalizes the glands and organs by reducing stress and bringing about harmony	• Creates homeostasis in the body
	• Advocates using tools for probing
	• Right foot represents the right side of the body; left foot, left side
• Is simple while bringing about amazing results	• Can correct specific problems and can treat and fix anything
• Can interpret the psychology of the client by reading their feet through foot conditions and structures (e.g. narrow steps indicate a narrow mind)	• Absolutely safe, can use it on everyone at anytime.
	• There are magic buttons on the feet corresponding to organs of the body
	• Doesn't know how it works, but it does

The statements above are taken from a review of literature. Authors of these statements offer no scientific validation of their hypotheses. In the following pages the objective is to apply critical thinking analysis and evaluate these statements from the scientific community's point of view.

Chart 1

statements and see how they stand up when scrutinized from the scientific community's point of view. This is not to be perceived as an attack, but rather an evaluation. Remember the crutch. The developer of the crutch would be proud of the advances in his creation if for no other reason than the benefits and comfort the design now provides to the patient.

• **Electro-chemical response.** This is quite plausible but the author does not continue on to tell how or why, or substantiate this claim with studies.

carry signals to the central nervous system. Some of these are triggered by special neurons called receptors which will be discussed in greater detail in Chapter 12. From a conventional physics point of view the synapse and how it functions—in essence, the 'solid' elements of the nerve—is the focus. In using a quantum physics perspective what happens in the spaces between the synapses—the dynamics of the 'silent gap' as Deepak Chopra refers to it—is of greater importance.

In Chapter 4 both the viewpoints of

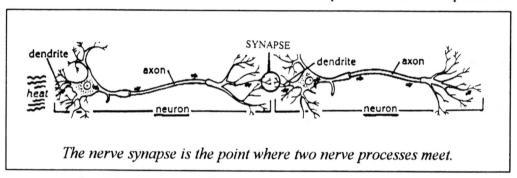

The nerve synapse is the point where two nerve processes meet.

• **Works through the nerve endings.** This statement is not anatomically correct. Nerves do not have endings as such. A nerve is a bundle of cells that carries signals. A single nerve cell is a neuron. A synapse is a junction between two neurons that allows one neuron to trigger an impulse in another. When a nerve impulse reaches the synaptic knob at the end of the axon (the long filament in a neuron), it triggers the release of a substance called a neurotransmitter. This crosses the gap between the two cells and begins a second neuron action. There is a special synapse between neurons and muscle fibers at the neuromuscular junction. When an impulse arrives at the synapse, it makes the muscle contract. Sensory neurons

Newtonian and quantum physics will be explored in greater detail.

• **Endorphin Release** - The concept has been taken out of a medical text. There is quite a body of literature on the release of endorphins, the body's natural pain killers, being activated by touch *anywhere* on the body. However, these studies are in relation to acupressure applied to the body. There are those who would take these results and conclude pressure applied to the feet will produce endorphin release. Nevertheless, this is conjecture. We must assess whether this claim is valid through research.

• **Unconscious response of the nervous system.** The nervous system is the center of communicative skills within the body. One author claims a reflex action is an involuntary or unconscious response to a stimuli. Though this is accurate, does it apply to working on the feet? How can a response of pressure to the feet be involuntary? It is voluntary to the point that the sensory nerves are being touched, so we have a voluntary activity. The reflexes or responses that are involuntary are unconscious responses. This is only true if you work on the autonomic nerve ganglia. There is an indirect pathway to the autonomic nervous system which must be considered, but this is limiting if it is the only consideration.

• **Autonomic Reflex.** Several authors speak about this. They may have drawn a correct conclusion, but they do not go far enough in explaining it or linking their theory to anything. Anatomically it is true that electrochemical nerve impulses set in motion pass through afferent neurons which carry messages into the center of the ganglia located outside of the spinal cord of the brain. From the ganglia, messages are taken by efferent neurons, those carrying messages out of the center to a specific organ which will then respond. This describes the body's autonomic nerve link-up, but the question remains, does this process occur when points on the feet are stimulated. Has research been conducted to validate this theory? Is any such mechanical response possible due to the complexity of the nervous systems?

• **Autonomic nerve reflex response stimulates internal organs, muscles and glands.** Three authors claim there's an autonomic reflex. Is this a thing, an object, or a specific physical

reflex unknown to science? Or are they talking about a response following a nerve pathway? These authors again do not link anything else to their statement as to how or why. No explanation is offered to their meaning.

• **Communication between the zones.** This concept brings up many questions. Has there been any investigation or scientific acceptance of the existence of zones? Is a zone a physical thing or an energy field, something similar to an acupuncture meridian? Will electromagnetic research bear out the existence of zones the way it has with acupuncture meridians? If they exist, does the nervous system communicate with the zones? To all of these questions there are currently no answers. More will be said about this concept of zones later in the chapter.

• **Locomotion/walking.** Is walking the same as having a foot therapy session? What if the person has biomechanical problems, how are all the zones or areas of the foot being stimulated?

• **Is a science, an art.** The term art has many meanings. Is the author talking about a skill, or practical application of knowledge, or one's creativity? Is a definition provided? What is the scientific basis? Where are the relevant scientific documents needed to sustain a 'science'?

• **Works through connective tissue massage, lymphatic drainage, autonomic nervous system and reflection.** This is a sensible statement. It implies that results of working on the feet affect several systems of the body and is all inclusive.

• **Produces relaxation and rest.** True, but the act of touching and caring produces relaxation. It has been written that reflexology promotes relaxation, assisting the body to heal itself and cleanse all systems of the body. How can a tactile therapy alone do this? It is now quite a valid theory that stress and the lack of the body's ability to relax is a contributing factor to many Western diseases. We can link Western disease statistics, that are readily available through university studies, with the stress factors which produce changes in physiology leading to disease. For instance one's profession has been linked to the probability of heart disease. One's personality type or lifestyle can lead to heart attacks. The question is: Is relaxation all that happens? It may be found that relaxation is an integral part of an enormous framework in which the practitioner works, but it is not the total picture.

• **Stress release.** Stress is a much abused word today. Research has shown that there is both positive and negative stress. Both kinds are needed for our existence. Does working on the feet selectively release only negative stress? What is negative and by whose definition? The stress reduction concept is another representation of the medical approach—one of treating a symptom. The response of the body *may be* to produce profound relaxation, but it may not. Rather than the use of the term stress reduction, tactile stimulation may be a more appropriate description of what happens. Touching the body in a caring way produces a relaxing or stimulating effect depending on the body's innate intelligence's assessment of what the body needs most at the time. When

this is combined with a willingness on the part of the client to succumb to the sensory stimulation an opportunity for healing occurs.

• **Energy systems/pathways/chi energy.** Meridians and acupuncture points have been proven to exist. During a foot therapy session very powerful meridians are affected. This is one reason why such profound results are achieved. There is an emphasis by some authors to concentrate on meridians and call the therapy reflexology. This causes confusion. There are many different types of energy and these should be defined, as much as possible, in the valid framework that presently exists and keep up with the literature in the field of the many energies that are currently being investigated. The question remains, does pressure to the feet work on or with these same points? Are these points identical to reflex points? Electrically are they the same or different? How can the acupuncture meridians be influenced and accessed by palpation of the feet? In what sequence should they be manipulated? How are results achieved?

According to Cerney[1] "Also finding its genesis in the foot is the kidney meridian. It's the only meridian on the bottom of the foot and begins underneath the foot just behind the third metatarsal head."[1] It should be noted that all other meridians that have points of entry and exit in the foot are located on the lateral, medial or dorsal aspects of the foot, not on the plantar surface where most of the practitioner's time is spent working.

• **Stimulates creativity and productivity.** Working the feet brings the body into balance and promotes creativity and productivity. How? Does that mean if I have my feet reflexed I will be able to draw? I cannot paint or draw now, but if I have my feet worked on it will stimulate my creativity and I will be an artist? What are the definitions of these terms?

• **Creates homeostasis in the body.** The word homeostasis is frequently misused. By medical definition, homeostasis is a tendency toward stability in the normal body states of the organism, it does not mean to help nature to normalize or balance. Homeostasis occurs without external stimulus—it is accomplished by the organs internally and individually by themselves. Practitioners do not bring the body into a state of homeostasis. Working on the feet is an external stimulus therefore, the internal response is not homeostatic.

• **Corrects specific problems; can treat and fix anything; is absolutely safe, can use it on everyone at any time.** These statements infer every condition can be diagnosed and treated safely. What about contraindications? Are there no contraindications? If there are no contraindications then it stands to reason that working on the feet cannot have any significant influence on any system of the body because if there is no action, then there is no reaction: no reaction, no contraindication. If in fact, there is significant benefit to health with the use of foot therapy, then there must be a physiological awareness about possible cautions and contraindications. Working on the feet provides the possibility of producing dynamic

results and should be respected accordingly

• **Can diagnose through the feet.** Several authors recommend medical intervention if their suggested treatment does not work, rather than referring the client to the doctor first before work begins. Is this in the client's best interest? Is this a legally safe practice? The inference that a sore spot on the foot indicates congestion to a particular organ is too restrictive and bears little credibility as the foot has not been considered in this equation. Pain anywhere indicates a problem to the immediate area which may indirectly affect other areas.

• **Is a simple method of producing balance.** It is simple in its application. Reflexology is non-invasive and can be performed anywhere at any time. Those are the luxuries of working on the feet. But we must be careful of the statement, "it's a simple thing; anyone can do it anywhere, it is safe for all conditions and there are no contraindications." The dynamics created are anything but simple and to date it is not known what they are and therefore discretion is called for. When a pathology is present, one must evaluate the presence of contraindications and proceed accordingly. We must be cautious about claims that may affect 'informed consent'.

• **Works by stimulating weak muscles.** This explanation is a half-truth and is too simplistic. Weak tissues in the feet—muscles, ligaments, and tendons—do decrease circulation. Tissue responds well to hands-on techniques, but this must be accompanied by sensible recommendations for strengthening exercises.

• **Is a form of massage.** Although linked in some ways and are complementary to each other, the techniques of massage and foot therapy are two separate disciplines. The fields have separate bodies of knowledge, histories, theories, definitions, scopes of practice, research, use distinct terminology, as well as different hands-on techniques.

• **Advocates using tools for probing.** Several authors recommend the use of tools. The moment we take the tactile approach away do we lose the best aspect of the therapy—touch? As a tactile therapy do we not need to touch our clients? It is generally believed that people need non-sexual, safe touch to flourish. Is endorphin release reduced when using tools? Do we lose the skill and sensitivity that is going to assist with our analysis? Can a tool assess tissue to the same degree as our hands can? If a tool breaks might we be inviting litigation? Worse still, do we run the risk of injuring our client? Is this not an important consideration for any profession?

• **Improves circulation.** Yes, palpation to the feet does *stimulate* the circulatory system. Improved peripheral vascular return is a primary result and *one* of the physiological responses.

• **Psychologically can interpret the life and mental health of the person by looking at the feet.** How is this possible? Does one come from a chemical, biomechanical and/or structural deviation point of view? What valid research is available to sustain this thought process? Is the basis of interpretation on empirical data or anecdotal stories being used as evidence? What are the ethical issues involved? Are the conclusions drawn from judgments on the practitioner's part? If so, what untold emotional harm could result from this?

Historically Baptista Pora, considered to be founder of physiognomy[2], was a man distinguished in his day for his attainments in science. In 1598 he published a folio entitled *De Human Physiognomia.* Later, in the 1880s and 90s, phrenology[3] and physiognomy were popular scientific studies and classified as branches of anthropology—the science of man. In essence they were contemplated to be the study of the relationship between the external and the internal. As Shakespeare wrote, " I do believe thee, I saw his heart in his face." Are authors attempting to apply this same concept to the feet? Does a physical problem always have to have an emotional cause or could it come from a biomechanical and structural basis? If emotional, where is the training or research for the therapist to do this kind of interpreting? What is the scope of practice? Are we infringing upon the professions of psychology, psychiatry, or psychotherapeutics? What are the ethical, moral and educational considerations?

Samuel R. Wells in his work *New Physiognomy*, (1894) quotes the famous physiognomist, Lavater as saying, "I understand but little of physiognomy, I have been and continue to be daily mistaken in my judgment..."[4] Is there a caution here for authors and practitioners attempting to apply this statement least they jump to conclusions and cause the client emotional harm?

The advocates of this judgmental style are neglecting what Dr. Larry Dossey (1993) in this text, *Meaning & Medicine* encourages all therapists to focus on: meaning and interpretation. The practitioners who address these two aspects in their therapy claim to treat the 'whole person'. Dossey states "...those health workers who most vigorously advocate treating the 'whole person' seem the most likely to neglect the importance of meaning."[5] He takes the challenge further and clearly focuses on mind/body paradigms. "One can, for instance, find numerous 'alternative' or 'holistic' health books replete with tables and formulae purporting to show that a physical problem in the patient's past—lack of parental love, child abuse, poor self-esteem, and an array of other deficiencies in nuturance and upbringing [is the cause]. ...What is left out of these simplistic notions, among other things is the unique, individual and idiosyncratic nature of meaning.

Dossey continues, "Because identical happenings in two different persons' lives may mean different things to each of them, it is impossible in principle to make rigid, uniform connections between life events and physical illness."

Apart from a psychological interpretation from looking at the client's feet, much can be gained from observation of the client. From a physiological perspective, a link can be observed between stance, posture gait cycle and psychology. A person's body stance does relate to a person's emotional state in the way they walk and stand. For instance, people who put weight on the forefoot may tend to be stooped shouldered, hold their head down and suffer from depression. When that is the case, they may not be toeing off properly during the gait cycle and therefore the reflexes to the cranial cavity are not being stimulated as they walk. Or the problem may stem from a weakness in the leg and thigh muscles and the knees with no abnormal psychological condition present. These clinical observations and deductions however are far from psychologically 'reading' the feet. The importance of clinical observation, a lost art today, will be discussed more fully in the next chapter.

• **Don't know how it works, but it works.** From the students' literature review it was found that some authors avoid putting forth any theories and simply state that the discipline works. Working on the feet should simply be accepted because it works.

Five Widely Accepted Statements

Let us take a moment to examine the five most widely accepted theories in further detail so that we might develop a greater understanding of the principles.

1. The foot houses objects known as reflexes that correspond to various body parts.

2. The body can be divided into ten zones of influence.

3. The shape of the medial aspect of the foot corresponds to the shape of the spine.

4. The entire body is mirrored on the feet.

5. Pressure applied to the feet will affect the function of the body by breaking down crystals or crystalline deposits.

Now, let us assess these key statements in more depth to discover whether or not they can be justified with the present knowledge of science today, or whether alternative principles exist which may be more applicable.

1. The foot houses objects known as reflexes that correspond to various body parts.

Reflexes are psychologically seductive. They allow the practitioner to appear wise and to have special insight into the client. Most practitioners and authors in the field of reflexology would define a reflex as an object. An object whose locations they are taught to memorize. It would certainly appear to be so based on the charts and tables. Yet, even with today's sophisticated and sensitive measuring devices we cannot prove a particular point or area on the foot is a reflex corresponding to a particular gland, organ or part of the body. The accuracy of isolating points to such an extent is questionable due to the complexity of how the body works and the overlapping tissue found in the foot and body. The success of the work may have nothing to do with reflex points. The application of pressure to the feet, whether specific or general in nature, does produce chemical, neurological and other changes in the body. This explains part of the process.

Today not everything is known about the body and how it functions. Much of it still remains a mystery. Science may eventually discover a new and separate reflex grid system of some kind, laid over the physical, which is composed of areas that provide treatment within an energy based concept. These may behave much like the acupuncture system of meridians which, though unseen, has been electromagnetically proven to exist, but it is doubtful one specific point will affect another specific area. Man is much more complicated and interconnected than that. Perhaps in studying the interconnectedness of the body, explanations may be found.

2. The body can be divided into ten zones of influence.

Dr. Ivan A. Tarasiok of Kiev studied with monks in a remote Chinese monastery in Siberia in the late 1960's. The monks were effectively treating patients with what Dr. Tarasiok termed reflexology. When interviewed, Dr. Tarasiok, speaking in Russian, indicated he was working on zones. Each time he used the word it was pronounced in English. He explained that a zone was simply an area of the body being worked on. The zone could be big or small, go across the body or up and down the body, it could be anywhere and could be a different area each time. He was correctly using the word in an anatomical context. His use of the word had nothing to do with zones dividing the body into ten longitudinal areas.

In another case, Russian doctor Natalia Bekhterev, director of Leningrad's Brain Institute, reports the pinpointing of two thousand zones of the brain, each having a different purpose.[6] Once again it would appear that the use of the word zone is being used in the proper medical context as an area under discussion.

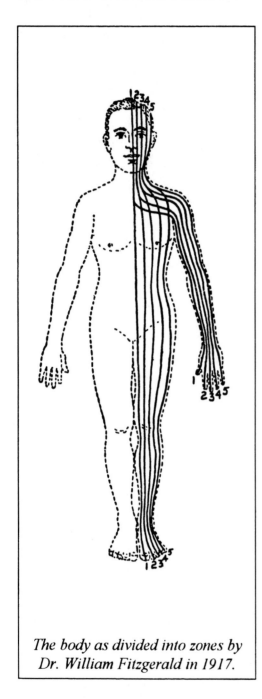

The body as divided into zones by Dr. William Fitzgerald in 1917.

This information leads one to wonder if Dr. Fitzgerald misunderstood the term he possibly heard about in Vienna and misused the term zone in his book. Or was this his attempt to simplify a concept for the public? After all, he was a doctor and would have been familiar with the correct term for zones. It is interesting to note that Fitzgerald drew straight lines down the body. Yet, in nature nothing is straight. For instance, natural barriers like mountains and rivers are not straight, lightning does not arc in a straight line. Only man draws arbitrarily straight lines to divide things. Even the meridians of Chinese Traditional Medicine are not found as straight lines. Alfons Cornelius' illustrations of painful areas published in Berlin in 1902 are not entirely straight either but appear to be more like meridians.[7]

It is important to achieve a happy medium between complexity and simplification in anatomy, if an explanation is too complex the explanation may be difficult and confusing; if over simplified, it may not be adequately definitive or may even be misleading. Unquestionably we do know that sagittal planes divide the body from top to bottom much like the zones described by Fitzgerald. And zones are used to define areas under discussion. We also know there is no definite number of sagittal planes which bisect the body, however, there is only one *medial* sagittal plane which is the center sagittal plane. Was Fitzgerald referring to sagittal planes but simplified the concept for the public?

3. The shape of the medial aspect of the foot corresponds to the shape of the spine.

Simply by observing and comparing the foot to the body it is clear the shape of the foot coincides with the shape of the body from the top of the head to the buttocks.

We know:

- the medial side of the foot is exactly the shape of our spine. There are four curves in the foot and four curves in the spine.

- These four divisions in the feet also correspond to the four body cavities. The hallux represents the cranial cavity; the metatarsals, the thoracic cavity; the tarsals equate to the abdominal cavity and the calcaneus to the pelvic cavity.

- With both feet together the back of the calcaneus is exactly the same shape as the iliac crest of the pelvic area.

- The calcaneus is the heaviest bone in the foot and the pelvic bones are the heaviest in the body.

- With both feet together, the heads of the metatarsals form the same shape as the diaphragm.

- When the great toe is turned sideways and bent in half at the first metatarsophalangeal joint, the same angle is observed as when the head is bent down. The shape of the distal phalanx is the same shape as from C1 to C7 [cervical 1 to cervical 7] in the neck.

- The proportion of the hallux to the rest of the foot is in the same proportion of the head to the body.

- There are twenty-six major bones in the foot; twenty-six bones in the skull and twenty-six bones in the spine.

- Leonardo daVinci when writing on the proportions of the human body observes, " The big toe is a sixth part of this foot...and it is similar to the space from the mouth to below the chin." Later he states, "The foot is of a size equal to that of the head of the man, that is to say, from below the chin to the highest point of the head."[8]

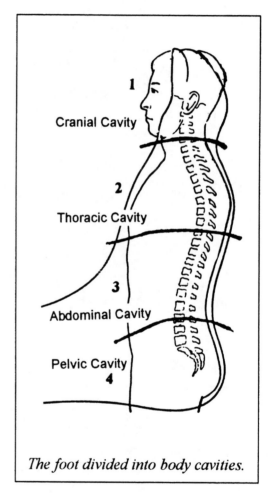

The foot divided into body cavities.

From these few indicators it would appear that the medial aspect of the foot corresponds to the shape of the spine. It also appears the shape of the foot is related to the head and trunk of the body.

Basically we are talking about the area from the top of the head to the buttocks. Once we want to find a point for the foot, or a foot reflex on the foot itself, or a knee reflex, or a reflex for the hands, we set up a questionable hypothesis. Even on the simplest level—that of visual observation—this theory cannot be validated.

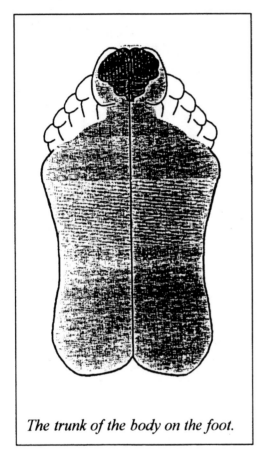

The trunk of the body on the foot.

On a more complex level there is no proof of a direct correlation between an area of the foot corresponding to an organ. This is a mechanical concept that bears no resemblance to fact. However, due to the influence of the autonomic nerve ganglia via pressure applied to the feet there is an indirect relationship. Additionally structural deviation from normalcy in the foot will set up torso stress that will affect organs generally.

4. The entire body is *mirrored* on the feet.

Rogers (1992) noted the mirror image and thought at the time that this concept was valid. However, applying critical thinking to the concept it became obvious this thought was not valid. A mirror image is a reversed image. This concept is in opposition to how charts are drawn. The correct terminology may be to say the feet house a somatic replication of the body, which has a wholistic focus. The somatic replication concept is not foreign to physiologists who recognize that each part of the body is represented by specific areas on the surface of the cortex of the brain known as the sensory homunculus and the motor homunculus. The more sensitive a particular part of the body is to stimuli, the greater is its area of the cortex as shown in the illustration on page 21.

Some writers use the term reiterated. Reiterated means repeat and the organ structure themselves are not repeated on the feet. Somatic replication means there is something in the foot which will stimulate an area in the body, not that the part is found on the foot as such.

Rather than say 'mirror image' the phrase, 'the body is reflected on the foot', is frequently used. However, to say the body is reflected on the foot is a very mechanical hypotheses and does not take into consideration the complex anatomy and physiology of the foot. Used as an illustration, this statement would explain the affects occurring elsewhere in the body when the foot is palpated. However, this is only one of a variety of explanations for how the foot can possibly represent the body.

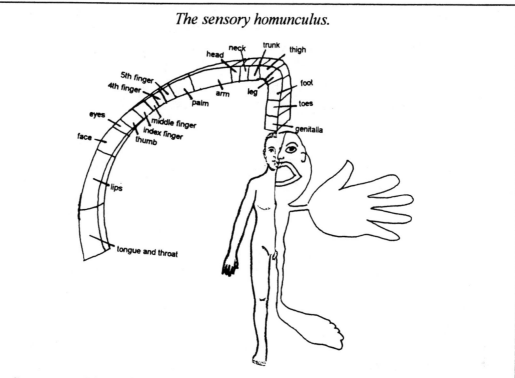

The sensory homunculus.

Sensations felt on the left side of the body are interpreted in the right sensory cortex of the brain and vice versa. Each part of the body is represented and if the body was drawn in proportion to the number of cells of the sensory cortex serving each part, it would look like the disproportionate figure on the right side.

Holograph

Another theory, related to the mirror image concept is the feet as a holographic unit. The hologram is a special three-dimensional picture created by energy interference patterns. It demonstrates a unique principle in nature which shows that every piece of something can contain the essence of the whole. The hologram provides us with a new and unique model which may help science to understand the structure of the body. This same holographic principle can be seen in the cellular structure of all living bodies. In the world of cellular biology every cell contains a copy of the master DNA blueprint or template of the entire human body.

Beyond the physical cellular level, other holographic units of the body exist in the energy field surrounding the human being. The first one is known as the *'etheric body'*. In metaphysical literature, it is said that the etheric body is one of many bodies contributing to the final expression of the human form. The etheric body, in all likelihood is an energy interference pattern similar to a hologram. The existence of the etheric body was first photographed by Semyon Kirlian in 1939. In the famous 'Phantom Leaf Effect' one third of a leaf was cut off and destroyed. Yet when electrophotographed the process recorded a whole leaf. It is thought by some scientists that the etheric body carries information for the growth, development, and repair of the physical body, while the genes with the DNA direct the molecular mechanisms governing the development of individual cells.[9]

Both the concepts of the hologram and somatic replication relate to the Eastern philosophy: 'as below, so above.' Or, the thought that the body is a microcosm of the macrocosm with man regarded as a miniature universe. Above the cellular level, is the foot a miniature replica of the body? Can we say, as *above* the foot, so *on* the foot?

Embryological Relationships

Another way of looking at the body is horizontally. Here the concepts of dermatomes and embryological development come into play. Embryology has proven that in the womb the human body grows not vertically but horizontally. In acupuncture, according to Mann (1973) when "...points on the kidney meridian are stimulated, they affect not only the kidney but also embryologically related organs such as the ovary, testicles, uterus, fallopian tube and, to some extent, the adrenal. This is because all these organs are formed in the same region of the embryo—the region of the kidney. This intimate relationship in the embryo is maintained in the adult, at least in so far as kidney acupuncture points are concerned."

Mann continues, "This, only one among hundreds of embryological relationships, is an example of how the interdependence of different parts of the body can be utilised in acupuncture."[10] This being so, we can ask ourselves: Is there a horizontal as well as vertical way that reflexology works? Historically, Dr. Joe Shelby Riley felt this was the case in 1924 when he divided the reflex zones on the feet in his book, *Zone Reflex*, both horizontally and vertically. Now it appears his concept can be verified using the latest in scientific research.

Chart Controversy

The question arises whether the holographic, embryological, or anatomical placement theories verify the placement of organ reflexes [providing that reflexes exist at all], on the many charts seen today. To date research in the field is almost always outcome based, and rarely focuses on the application or mechanisms by which the therapy works. The lack of scientific standards regarding charts leaves the studies, which have been performed thus far in question, not the outcomes. Work on the feet does affect the body, and in a very positive way. However, because no chart has been scientifically validated as accurate—i.e., that the placement of reflexes is accurate and a connection to the organs as claimed has been demonstrated—this lack of standardization results in another problem. One of the tenets for a study to be valid is that the results must be duplicable. In order to hope to duplicate results the same charts must be used. With no standardization of charts, what if a researcher uses a different chart? Or what if practitioners refer with one another about clients and they are not using the same chart? These questions are especially important if one is working or researching in the medical model—that is proving a certain medical condition is helped with the application of pressure to specific areas on the feet. When we speak of working in the relaxation model, which involves a more wholistic paradigm and is also very effective, it is possible to do so without any charts—in this case we are working with people, not conditions or specific areas on the foot, but the entire foot.

Conducting research which confirms or denies the application of pressure or mechanisms through which a method works is not as exciting as proving that a certain percentage of research subjects get relief from specific complaints. It also involves a threat to those who have devised charts. However, if we are going to have any credibility with the academic fields, research must begin at the beginning with objective research that is open to proving organ reflex placement and the results that are obtained with pressure. The field cannot afford to be blinded by biases and history. This kind of research must form the basis of all future research and chart standardization.

5. **Pressure applied to the feet affect the function of the body by breaking down crystals or crystalline deposits.**

Ingham (1951) writes, "At the *present time* [emphasis by Rogers & Issel] the assumption is that this tenderness is caused by the irritation of crystalline deposits in the area of the nerve reflex of any affected part...."[11] With the anatomical discoveries made over the last fifty years is it not time this concept be re-evaluated? Today several authors still use the term 'crystals'. An orthodox health care professional does not know about 'crystals'. He will tell you he has observed autopsies and has never seen a crystal in the feet. Crystals are formed elsewhere in the body and are clearly defined and named.

'Crystals' may be descriptive

of what the therapist is feeling to some extent, however, there is complex anatomy to feel with the thumb and fingers. The use of the word 'crystals' does not provide a proper definition to the underlying pathology as these substances felt can be defined using logical and anatomical terms.

The action of nerves does not literally end. Nerves come close together at synaptic points where the afferent and efferent nerves transmit messages. These are message receptors, not endings. (See page 11.) The application of pressure does produce a physiological change by sending a message via the afferent nerves which in turn transmits a message via the efferent neuron that conducts impulses away from the brain or spinal cord. Actually the space between the nerve synapses is so fine, a grain of baby powder cannot fit there, let alone a crystal. Yes, something may feel like a crystal or a grain of sand, but what is it we really feel?

One of the explanations for the gritty or grainy feeling experienced by the practitioner is the presence of adhesions. An adhesion is a scar that forms between two soft tissue structures as a result of injury. The injury could be the result of a cut, burn, contusion, stretching or tearing like a sprain or strain, repetitive movement, or chronic postural stress. The scar tissue is made up of fibrous tissue which commonly occurs between tendons or ligaments and bone and fills the empty space in damaged soft tissue.

Another word to describe the phenomena is 'lesion'. Leon Chaitow (1988) quotes Peter Lief's description of a lesion being formed by the following four causes:

1. Congestion of the local connective tissues

2. Disturbance of the acid-base balance of the connective tissues

3. Fibrous infiltrations [also known as adhesions]

4. Chronic muscular contractions or hyper-hypotropic [tone] changes

Lief goes on further to explain the causes which bring about muscular tensions. He sites:

1. Fatigue, exhaustion, bad posture

2. Local trauma

3. Systemic toxemia—the lack of exercise and oxygen

4. Dietetic deficiencies and

5. Psychosomatic causes

The presence of a lesion, he contends, is always revealed by an area of hypersensitivity to pressure.[12]

Chaitow (1988) quotes Brian Youngs, D.O. who uses much the same vocabulary, in describing the changes which are palpable in muscles and soft tissues associated with reflex effects as 'congestion'. "This ambiguous word can be interpreted as a past hypertrophic fibrosis. Reflex cordant contraction of the muscle reduces the blood flow through the muscular tissue and in such relatively anoxic regions of low pH and low hormonal concentration, fibroblasts proliferated and increased fibrous tissue is formed. This results in an increase in the thickness of the existing connective tissue partitions—the epimysia and perimysia—and also this condition probably infiltrates deeper between the muscle fibres to affect the normal endomysia. Thickening of the fascia and subdermal connective tissue will also occur if these structures are similarly affected by a reduced blood flow. Fat may be deposited, particularly in endomorphic types, but fibrosis is most pronounced in those with strong mesomorphic components—a useful pointer for both prognosis and prophylaxis."

Young continues, "Fibrosis seems to occur automatically in areas of reduced blood flow, e.g., in a sprained ankle—where swelling is marked and prolonged, in the lower extremities where oedema of any origin has been constant over a period.... Fibrous tissue can then take the strain instead of the muscle fibres. It is this long-term homeostatic reflex which apparently operated in all cases of undue muscle contraction, whether due to strain or tension."[13]

Judging from the above information it is now time to move away from the use of past vocabulary of crystals and crystalline deposits to more appropriate terminology like adhesion or lesion.

All disciplines spring from earlier professions or thoughts which congeal in a new form, take a broader perspective, or narrow into a specialty. These advances can only occur if the practitioners are willing to question each and every facet of their subject of study. One of the disciplines evolving from foot work is reflexognosy. While similar to reflexology it differs in its model., philosophy and its belief system. It begins by questioning some of the basic hypotheses of reflexology and incorporates other foot therapies. To this new field of study we shall now turn.

[1] Cerney, J.V. *Acupressure: Acupuncture without Needles*, Simon & Schuster, New York, NY 1974, pg. 35.

[2] Physiognomy is the practice of attempting to judge character and mental qualities by observation of bodily facial features.

[3] Phrenology is the practice of character analysis based on the study of the shape of the skull.

[4] Wells, Samuel R. *New Physiognomy*, Fowler & Wells Co, New York, 1894, pg 27.

[5] Dossey, Larry. *Meaning & Medicine*, Bantam Books, New York, 1993, pg. 15.

[6] Gris, Henry and William Dick. *The New Soviet Psychic Discoveries*, Prentice-Hall, Englewood Cliffs, New Jersey, 1978, pg 272.

[7] For an illustration of Cornelius' findings and the history of Fitzgerald's work see *Reflexology: Art, Science & History*.

[8] DaVinci, Leonardo. *Leonardo On Painting*, edited by Martin Kemp, Yale University Press, New Haven, 1989, pgs. 126-127.

[9] Ostrander & Schroeder. *Psychic Discoveries Behind the Iron Curtain*, Prentice Hall, Inc. Englewood Cliffs, NJ 1971, pg. 216.

[10] Mann, Felix. *Acupuncture, The Ancient Chinese Art of Healing and How it Works Scientifically*, Vintage Book, New York, 1973, pg. 40.

[11] Ingham, Eunice. *Stories the Feet Have Told*, Ingham Publishing, St. Petersburg, Florida, USA, 1951, pg. 15.

[12] Chaitow, Leon. *Soft Tissue Manipulation*, Healing Arts Press, Rochester, Vermont, 1988, pg. 34.

[13] Ibid. pg. 76.

Chapter 3

Reflexognosy™

**It is only with the heart that one can see rightly;
what is essential is invisible to the eye.**
—Antoine de Saint Exupery

Reflexology is traditionally defined as a combination of the words: *reflex* (a non-medical definition designating an involuntary reaction resulting from a stimulus) and *ology* (the study of this reaction).

Reflexognosy on the other hand takes a broader view. In this case *reflex* means to direct back through. *Ognosy* is taken from the Greek root *cognosy* meaning knowledge of; knowledge of what is directed back through the body from the feet. This allows one to explore a subject from all points of view. A clear example of the use of these suffixes can be found in pharmacology. Pharmacology is the science dealing with the preparation and use of drugs. While pharmacognosy is the science that deals with medicinal products of plant, animal, or mineral origins in the crude or unprepared state, their natural occurrence and historical use, as well as their use, and manufacture today. Both are concerned with the effects of drugs

on living organisms. The first is strictly a technical approach and the second a broader and more inquiring approach—literally looking at the subject from all points of view.

Reflexognosy is defined as the application of appropriate pressure to the legs and feet by the hands of a trained practitioner to bring about physiological and psychological changes stimulating subtle energies. It centers on whole health management of the person. Reflexognosy is not a new way of doing reflexology. It is a new way of theoretically approaching the understanding of the body and healing in general using the legs and feet. Its theories are drawn from ancient cultures, quantum physics, and various energy medicines. On the technique level it embraces podiatry, biomechanics, and soft tissue management with joint activation for energy stimulation. In dealing with anatomy and physiology it takes a new perspective from the concept of body cavities and how the anatomy housed within is affected by the way we walk. Through scientific research reflexognosy conclusively proves that body cavities are affected as we walk. The application of appropriate pressure to the feet and legs to facilitate a healing response within the client can produce the most astounding results. The practitioners who wish to develop a wholistic focus in their work find this broader viewpoint encouraging and complementary to their central discipline. Reflexognosy should not be seen to replace reflexology as it draws its theoretical base from many areas of study.

A Wholistic Approach

Reflexognosy studies the energetic characteristics of healing. There is no denying that the practitioner does not do the healing—that is left up to the innate intelligence and healing process of each body. The client by placing confidence in the therapy stimulates the direction of the healing responses on the physical, emotional, spiritual and innate intelligence levels. However, one of the roles of the practitioner is to create an environment in which healing can take place. Any man or woman who endeavors to practice a wholistic therapy by providing the opportunity for healing on all levels of being, physical, emotional, intellectual and spiritual, must be more than a good technician. To arrive at an understanding of the factors which may be involved with the client's complaint, the practitioner has to use faculties involving his intuition and listen to what the client's body is telling him, not only what the client may be verbalizing. The practitioner, while withholding judgment, must be a good listener and confidant, working according to the unique needs of the individual. The client benefits from intuitive insights that the wholistic practitioner has the ability to bring forth consciously or unconsciously.

The philosophical elements contained in this book are intended to help reflexognosists begin to add this area of study to their field without overwhelming them. Practitioners must be trained to add new meaning and assist to interpret responses on multiple levels. In reflexology one can find numerous formulae purporting to tell us where to work for certain physical conditions. Past literature written by Rogers (1992) looked at the concepts of feet in this way. Once academic rigor and debate were applied to the subject a shift took place from the mechanical view to a more wholistic view and detailed questions arose pertaining to the mechanism by which results were achieved. Rogers, when being questioned about this shift in thought stated, "I too was blinded by results. What is left out of these simplistic formulae is the concept that each human being is a complex, multifaceted individual and no two people will have the exact same cause of illness—be that on the physical, mental or emotional levels. When we practice with this formulae we are practicing in the medical model of treating symptoms, or focusing on the parts, not the whole. Then there is no opportunity to place meaning or any interpretation to the process." We treat the condition, not the person.

Reflexognosy works with the age old and nearly lost art of observation. Observation of the many structural and functional contributions that may be influencing the feet and legs, which in turn, may influence the rest of the body. This scientific aspect of the work is balanced by an intuitive approach. Because we seek to help our clients on all levels it is wise to speak both to their intellect and to their soul, or psyche, with these two aspects of our own being. In working with our clients we want to remember that although their minds ask for explanation and description, the rest of their being is seeking a *feeling* of connection and compassion. Reflexognosy brings this balance. It is a wholistic and dialectical approach—wholistic because it endeavors to treat the whole client, rather than address a complaint; dialectical, because it is held that the physical body is composed and influenced by non-material forces. Therefore the reflexognosist works with both the seen and the unseen. For as Antoine de Saint Exupery (1971) says in his wonderful book, *The Little Prince*, "It is only with the heart that one can see rightly; what is essential is invisible to the eye."[1]

The goal of reflexognosy is to develop a new occupation in the health field. The body of knowledge for this profession is based on the link between the feet and the body; physiologically what occurs during a session; the mechanisms by which results are achieved; the link between structural deviation from normalcy in the feet and disease states; plus preventive and corrective solutions to any structural deviation found—for deviation in structure precedes deviation in function. The working of reflexognosy can be explained through the sciences of anatomy, physiology and biomechanics blended

with energy medicine, and the skills of observation and palpation.

Palpation is a combination of touch, feel, examination, sensory feedback, and interpretation through experience. It involves proficiency in receiving specific information from touching the client. Palpation is not just a touching, however, but the art of sensing tissue changes in tension, temperature, dampness, movement, and swelling. Time and practice are needed to develop the skill of receiving information through manual contact. The reflexognosist learns to feel and interpret what is felt and observed.

The Importance of Clinical Observation

One of the most essential requirements in clinical practice is to develop observational skills. Observation by the practitioner is the bases of natural medicine systems like Traditional Chinese Medicine, Ayurvedic Medicine, Homeopathy, and Herbal Medicine. Observation of the clues given by the client's external body can reveal to the experienced practitioner much about what is going on with the client that the client may or may not even be aware of.

Observation does not mean judgment. It is an evaluation that may direct you to *possible* problems and ways of working with the client. Reflexognosists do this already when they observe the condition of the foot before they begin work. But we need to keep in mind that as practitioners we do not have the right to judge and state that anything we observe is a factual analysis. We are not doctors. It is not our responsibility to diagnose, but we can use our observational skills to decide if a referral to another practitioner is warranted. In addition, when dealing with the human body we need to keep in mind that nothing can ever be set in concrete as there are too many variables.

However, as the world is turning more and more to the natural therapist we must become eclectic in our approach and develop basic skills that have been given to us which include the power of observation. Our ability to observe our clients in a wholistic fashion will make us more effective practitioners. Observation can provide clues as to areas or systems of the body to emphasize during a session.

Observations include consideration of the client's general appearance, gait, attitude, speech, and much more. Observations here shall be confined to the physical aspect of the client that begins as soon as the person walks into the clinic. The following list is provided as a guide for what to look for during the consultation process.

Observations can tell the practitioner many things that are worth considering and noting on the client's record. The list on the following pages is only a guide. Don't jump to conclusions! Or blurt out something to the client. Observations must be supported by the client's history, and our tactile skills. Remember there is a person behind your observations. Making astute observations does require some training and practice. Just as the development of our tactile skills came through practice, so observational skills will come the more we use them.

In utilizing the expertise of observation there is a balance between the seen and unseen. Concentrating

upon a rational approach and observing the signs presented by the client, reflexognosists gradually enhance their intuitive powers of observation while combining this with reasoning faculties to come to a balanced judgment.

The foot and leg are the areas of focus for the reflexognosist and the surface upon where our hands-on work is applied. The reflexognosist must be educated to recognize and observe:

- the role of the feet and legs in health

- the way they act—the way they move

- the bones, joints and other tissues that are located in the feet

- the diseases which may effect them, and

- perform a full examination of the mechanism and intelligence of the lower extremities.

In essence the entire surface upon which the therapy is applied and the body which is attached to it, the dynamics which houses the anatomy, the unseen energy elements, and clinical observations are all of concern to the reflexognosist.

There are exciting new horizons for reflexognosists to explore as they set about to prove the validity and effectiveness of their chosen discipline. A powerful discipline. The feet and legs provide useful information as part of professional assessment if the practitioner only has eyes to see and hands to feel. They also provide the client a key to healing.

Observation	Possible indication of:
I. Gait Analysis:	
Rigidly	Fluidity in movement means much less tension throughout the entire body
Position of the head	If the head is straight and not bent toward the floor there is a good chance that the client has a positive approach to life. This is not judgment. This information comes from the pressure that develops from the head being carried forward. The anterior lobe of the brain, when under pressure is a contributing factor in states of depression.
Position of the shoulders	If the shoulders are rounded there will be pressure and tension on the thoracic cavity lessening the ability to breathe correctly and in turn lowering the ability of the body to carry the blood to the brain. Conditions that may be affected by rounded shoulders include asthma, bronchitis, upper respiratory infections, and lowered resistance.
Do the knees bend	The knees when bent during locomotion lessen the tension in the skeletal framework and the supporting musculature.
Do the hips move	An easy gait pattern gives the appearance of a rolling and easy flowing action from the hips. This flowing appearance gives the body the fluidity that it needs to avoid rigidity. Also, if the thigh and hip do not turn, the gait is thrown off and one waddles like a duck. The heavy musculature of the buttocks and thighs if not used properly diminishes the flow of blood through the large arteries—the femoral common iliac—to the legs and feet. This can contribute to peripheral vascular disability.
Is there a spring in the step	When present the shock absorption of the feet and the discs are working. To what degree can only be determined by a professional examination.
Shuffling, dragging gait	A dragging look within the gait phase gives the clue that there may be muscle and skeletal problems. Additionally there may be problems within joints, restricting movement. The person may have low energy and pain.
When Seated:	
Moves around, uncomfortable	Not at ease, may be due to many factors. Never come to conclusions without drawing the client into the discussion. Talk slowly and ask if there is

Observation	Possible indication of:
When Seated:	
Moves around, uncomfortable (continued)	anything s/he would like to add. Give ample time for a response. Talk slowly and watch for the client to be come settled.
Crosses and uncrosses legs	Can be nervousness, if so adopt the above suggestion. It can also be linked to rigidity factors in the body. This observation may be linked to earlier observations made during the walking phase.
Shuffling of feet	Can be due to painful joints or lower back disturbance or agitation
Crossing feet	Infers discomfort in the skeletal framework. Wanting to stretch and cross legs even after a short time sitting may suggest that stretching be incorporated into any part of therapy or homework.
II. Appearance of Feet	
Skin:	
Pale	Circulation may need to be stimulated.
Purple	Stimulation needed to the circulation.
Blue	Poor circulation, low energy.
Redness	Excess circulation; or poor venous return.
Odorous	Toxic condition; check for assimilation/elimination problems.
Peeling	Mineral deficiencies; footwear not allowing foot to breathe, systemic or local infection.
Cracked and dry heels	Trauma from footwear—the footwear is absorbing the oils from the feet making them crack; chickweed ointment can be applied.
Cold	Poor circulation; low energy; alertness low.
Hot spots	Nervous system may be a factor; or hormone imbalance.
Rigid	Tension throughout the body.
Dorsiflexed at the ankle or toes	Overactivated leg muscles; tension.
One foot falling in and the other out when lying down	Hip socket or muscles tight, exercises for hips to be given.
Corns	Shoes too short or too narrow.
Callous	Dry friction from shoes, wearing high heels, having a bone out of place, improper gait. A callous on the medial side of the hallux indicates dry pressure and friction to that area and places tension on the neck and shoulders during locomotion.

Observation	Possible indication of:
Swelling around the ankles	Trauma and scar tissue build-up from sprains, hormone imbalance, elimination or cardiac problems must be considered.
Scars	Trauma, extra sensitivity.
Moles	Watch closely for any sudden changes.
Warts	Viral condition.
Rash	Possible tinea, excema, or contact dermatitis—an irritation caused by environmental factors such as soaps, nylons, dye in shoes.
Thick or heavy hair growth	Hormone imbalance.
Sore that doesn't heal	Diabetes.
Cracked nails	Nutritional; minerals required.
Yellowed and thick nails	Fungus.

III. General Appearance:

Eyes

Bright & Clear	Indicates good health as they have a direct link to the Central Nervous System.
Whites Clear	Good oxygenation usually.
Marked iris	The iris offers constitutional information. If there is a white ring round the iris this usually indicates there has been a major emotional upset, shock or trauma at sometime.
Yellowing in the eye	Infers toxic system. In this case be slow and patient with the therapy. Encourage the body slowly to accept the healing stimulus you are using. Stimulation too quickly can be far too much for this person. Lighter pressure may be appropriate.

Skin

Dry	May be hormonal condition or diet. Light olive oil introduced into the diet in small monitored amounts may be of assistance.
Cracked	As above. Also consider the inclusion of minerals.
Prematurely aged	Hormones may be an influence as well as diet. A wholistically trained nutritional practitioner will be of assistance here.

Mouth

Tight	Indicates facial tension—facial/scalp massage may be considered.

Observation	Possible indication of:
Mouth (continued) Dry	Saliva is a powerful laxative, a dry mouth may be the reason for constipation or sluggish elimination. The introduction of bitters into the diet will stimulate saliva production. One way of promoting bitters is to eat dandelion leaves which are also good for the liver and gallbladder
Lips	
Healthy color	Indication that circulation to the head is adequate
Pale	Indicates lack of oxygen. Stimulating circulation may help
Cracked	Dry mouth and lack of saliva. Follow instructions for dry Mouth
Tongue	Examination useful for constitutional indication and usually indicates the overall functioning of the gastro-intestinal tract.
Coated	If due to dry mouth demonstrates an inability to assimilate and eliminate correctly. See addition of bitters in diet given above. Inclusion of minerals will also be of benefit. Consult wholistically trained nutritional practitioner to assist in determining which minerals may be useful.
Yellow	Needs potassium sulfate.
White	Needs potassium chloride.
Brown/mustard colored	Needs potassium phosphate.
Hands	
Relaxed	At ease and comfortable.
Wringing	Uneasy.
Skin dry and cracked	Diet, hormones, environmental considerations. Castor oil baths helpful
Clammy	Nervous.
Nails	Can indicate diet or medication needs to be addressed.
Cracked, soft and/or peeling	Needs calcium.
Bitten	Nervous agitation.
Chipped	Broad base of minerals needed.
Breathing	
Easy and deep	Calm, settled.
Shallow and uneven	Oxygenation factor to be considered.
Shallow only	Lesson on breathing to aid oxygenation and energy level to be given.
Sighing	Diaphragm compression.

Observation	Possible indication of:
Face/Complexion	
Grey	Lack of oxygen, illness, exhaustion.
Rosy	Good oxygen.
Pale	Lack of oxygen, tired, weary.
Acne/skin eruptions	Elimination factors, hormones, diet to be considered.
Ears	
Color matches face	Good circulation.
Red around edges	Uneven circulation.
Pale to face	Low circulation.
Blue	Bad circulation.
Dry and scaly	Environmental, circulatory, and diet to be considered.
Speech	
Clear, strong voice	Positive attitude, relaxed.
Quiet and uncertain	Unsure, needs encouragement.
Ranting	Emotional uncertainty.
Rambling	Nervous; confused.
Evasive	Lack of positive approach to treatment.
Hair	
Shining	Overall good balance.
Dull	Circulation, diet and elimination slow.
Thinning, or dry & brittle	Mineral deficiency, lack of assimilation.
Oily	Check diet for oils and fats, assimilation/elimination sluggish.

The following three chapters will deal with the subject of energy. This discussion will assist reflexognosists in developing their philosophical base and bring a new understanding of the human being that can be applied to their work.

---

[1] de Saint Exupery, Antoine. *The Little Prince*, Harcourt Brace Jovanovich, Publishers, San Diego, 1971, pg. 87.

Chapter 4

Energy—The New Frontier

It is possible there exists human emanations that are still unknown to us. Do you remember how electrical currents and 'unseen waves' were laughed at? The knowledge about man is still in its infancy.

—Albert Einstein

Rossi (1994) in his introduction to the text, *Mind-Body Therapy* offers advice that bears relevance to reflexognosists. Drawing from his ideas, we as practitioners should look to recent data released through podiatry, osteopathy, energy medicine, and quantum physics as this information may enable the 'true believing' clinician or the skeptical laboratory researcher to join hands in a united effort to create a new science for reflexognosy. Rossi joins, 'mind-body-healing'[1] as a combination. This is the same approach that professional reflexognosists are wishing to combine.

Energy is a word that is tossed about frequently and to most people's minds is associated with 'New Age' mysticism or the chi of Oriental medicine. Because of this association, the term energy is often, in Western circles, given little credibility. In spite of how confus-ing the word is, it has validity in all cultures, even in Western societies.

The word energy stems from the Greek word *ergon*, meaning work. Energy, in scientific terms, is defined as a power that may be translated into motion, overcoming resistance, or effecting physical change; the ability to do work. In physics it is the capacity to perform work. Energy assumes several forms. It may be thermal in the form of heat, electrical, mechanical, chemical, radiant, nervous, potential, psychic, and nuclear to name but a few manifestations. In doing 'work', the energy is changed from one form to another or to several forms.

Scientifically, *potential* energy refers to that energy in existence that is not being exerted at the time. *Electrical* energy is concerned with the flow of electrons and how the flow can create work. This in turn, when moving in a stream as electrical current, gives rise to a *magnetic* field of force with which *kinetic* energy, or the energy of motion, is associated. *Mechanical* energy on the other hand is the part of physical science which treats the laws of motion and the effect of forces upon the working of machines. *Free* energy is the energy equal to the maximum amount of work that can be obtained from a process occurring under conditions of fixed temperature, pressure and volume.

Probably one of the most notorious forms of energy is *nuclear* or *atomic* energy. Atomic theory states that all material objects and substances are composed of atoms, and that various phenomena are explained by the properties and interactions of these atoms. Energy is given off in the course of nuclear reaction by changes in the nucleus of an atom through fission.

Radiant energy is the energy contained in light rays or any other form of radiation like sunlight. In ordinary light, rays of energy move randomly in many directions at once. However, in the laser this energy is organized into an orderly beam producing a powerful energetic effect.

While a number of different kinds of energy have been mentioned here, it is well to remember that scientists do not know what energy really is. They are able to measure its effect, and can usually agree upon the results. Nevertheless what energy exactly is remains a mystery. However, we do not have to 'see' energy in order to believe in its existence or its effect. Science, led by quantum physics is evolving into a new understanding of energy.

A Shift in Paradigm

According to Webster's New World Dictionary, paradigm is defined as: 1. a pattern, example, or model; 2. an overall concept accepted by most people in an intellectual community, as a science, because of its effectiveness in explaining a complex process, idea or set of data. A vision of a new reality brought about through a fundamental change in our thoughts, perceptions, and values leads to a shift in paradigm.

Such profound cultural transformations do not take place very often and when they do occur they affect every level of society, from individuals, to governments, to economics and culture. In discussing scientific revolutions, Thomas Kuhn in his book *The Structure of Scientific Revolutions* shows that almost every significant breakthrough in the field of science is first a break with tradition, with the old ways of thinking and with old paradigms. For instance to Ptolemy, the Egyptian astronomer, the earth was the center of the universe. But Copernicus took a different interpretation and said the sun was the center of our universe. Whenever a shift in paradigm is called for it is usually met with a great deal of resistance and persecution for the revealer of the new found truth. The paradigm that is now shifting has dominated our culture for 400-500 years and is associated with the Scientific Revolution of the 16th & 17th centuries, the Industrial Revolution, beginning about 1760, and the Age of Enlightenment in the 18th century. It is a belief in Sir Isaac Newton's view of the universe. This antiquated paradigm includes the belief in:

1. The scientific method as the only valid approach to knowledge

2. The universe and everything in it as a mechanical system composed of elementary material building blocks

3. Unlimited material progress through economic and technological growth with little thought to its impact on our natural resources and nature.

The new paradigm based on the work of Einstein and his colleagues involves the belief that:

1. The rational and intuitive are complementary modes of functioning of the human mind, both being given equal weight, with acknowledgment of the body/mind connection

2. Structure is determined by process. The dynamic processes of movement and energy are studies, not necessarily the end results

3. Includes a reverence for all living organisms and a belief that everything is interconnected.

In order to understand the shift in paradigm which is occurring, one needs to look at the basis of and for the shift, how it came about and then narrow the view to how it does and will impact the field of reflexognosy.

The Age of Scientific Revolution began with the philosophy and mathematics of Descartes (1596-1650), the father of analytic geometry, which was quickly followed by the mathematical genius of Newton (1642-1727) who gave the world differential calculus. According to Descartes, mind and body belonged to two parallel but fundamentally different realms, each of which could be studied without reference to the other. Descartes wrote, "There is nothing in the concept of body that belongs to mind; and nothing in that of mind that belongs to the body." The body he decided was governed by mechanical laws—and because there was no purpose, life, or spirituality in matter, it could be explained in terms of the arrangement and movement of its parts—it was simply a machine. Descartes is responsible for the splitting of the mind and body, however in all fairness he did believe in the mind—or soul—which he theorized as being free and immortal. He believed the soul was clearly and specifically identified with consciousness and could affect the body by interacting through the brain's pineal gland. It was later scientists who deleted any mention of the soul.

In essence, Newton's theories of physics was built on the principle of the assemblage of parts. Newtonian physics is called reductionism—to reduce things to their smallest unit [originally cells] that can be seen and measured—later in the 1950s this expanded, thanks to the development of molecular biology, to include molecules. Classical Newtonian physics provided medicine with a working view of illness based on the concept of a mechanical clockwork like body that keeps on running unless there is a mechanical breakdown through disease. The body is seen as a machine that can be dismantled and reduced into smaller and smaller parts.

> **The Body As a Mechanical Machine**
>
> - **The heart as a pump**
> - **The lungs as bellows**
> - **The joints as gears and levers**
> - **The nervous system as electrical circuitry**
> - **The brain as a computer**
> - **The eye as a camera**
> - **The stomach as a chemical beaker**
> - **The intestines and urinary tract as plumbing**
> - **The liver and kidneys as filters**

This model largely ignores the possible influence of the mind and consciousness on the functioning of the human body. Because the human body is primarily regarded as material or a physical object, and reduced to a series of replaceable parts repaired by drugs and surgery, this very mechanical and technological viewpoint is understandable.

If Newton's theories had been correct then the deeper one penetrates into the mysteries of nature, the more mechanical or predictable things should become and act. Going from the organ to the cell, events move mechanically and logically. Things react the same way when you go from the cell to the molecule. But this theory has now been found to be partial or incomplete. With the scientific strides that have been made at the beginning of the 20th century, Newton's theory has its limitation. Atoms combine to form molecules. They consist of a complex arrangement of electrons revolving about a positively charged nucleus containing [except for hydrogen] protons and neutrons and other particles. At the beginning of this century, with the scientific advances that were made by Einstein and other physicists, much higher predictive and explanatory values were provided.

Quantum Physics

According to *Stedman's Medical Dictionary*, "energy can also be defined as a dynamic force."[2] Dynamic force is something physicists study, and just as with other professions, the field of physics has struggled in its professional growth and development to accept the new and completely different way of looking at how the world operates in quantum physics.

Quantum physics is the branch of physics that studies the energetic characteristics of matter at the subatomic level. It deals not so much with material things, but with fields of energy, with this dynamic force within objects. The new theories put forward by several of the physicists at the beginning of this century have actually stood the test of time. Yet, like other fields, there are many scientists who are resistant to change in spite of the

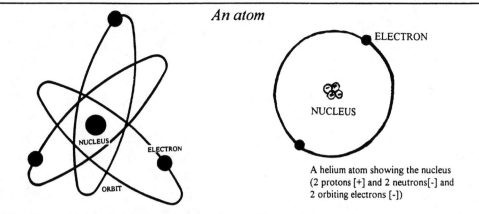

An atom

ELECTRON

NUCLEUS

A helium atom showing the nucleus
(2 protons [+] and 2 neutrons[-] and
2 orbiting electrons [-])

NUCLEUS

ELECTRON

ORBIT

The orbit is the path followed by electrons. Electrons are negative charged particles of electricity in the orbit. The nucleus is a compact mass of protons (+ positive charged particles) and neutrons (- negative charged particles). The Newtonian physicist investigates the orbit, electrons and nucleus—the 'solid' elements of the atom. The Quantum physicist looks at the spaces and the dynamics of this space within the nucleus which is the bonding power holding the nucleus together.

evidence.

Two contemporaries of Einstein's, Max Plank and Neils Bohr, help fill in some of the gaps of Eintein's theories. Bohr discovered the dual nature of electrons. They behave both as particles, that is as objects, and then as unseen waves of energy. Whether electrons are seen or unseen depends upon the design of the experiment. If the experiment was designed to prove that atoms are physical then that was the results the researcher got. If on the other hand one wanted to prove that particles were invisible and could be seen only by the pattern of energy they produced, one got that result. Electrons become like the wind, unseen, but their effect can be seen, felt, and measured.

With this breakthrough the dividing line in nature between the seen and the unseen becomes almost impossible to define. 20th century physics has shown that if one subdivides any one molecule,

further reduction in the size begins to reveal its unpredictable nature. Beyond the level of the molecules predictability becomes less mechanical. One enters into the world of quantum, a world governed by probability, unpredictable action, and in one word, energy.

Quantum physics acknowledges the interplay of numerous energetic forces which combine to form a whole. In this light the human being is basically a dynamic process and health is harmony of this movement, a movement of all the dynamic processes going on in the body at any one time in response to its internal and external environments. And we are a dynamic process, it has been proven that 98% of 120^{28} of the atoms that are found in the body are replaced annually. It is staggering that we have all that going on in us! Yet physically and mentally we appear to be solid, constant and unchanged for extended periods of time.

Quantum physics states that

every atom is more than 99% empty space and that sub-atomic particles moving at lightning speed are really just bundles of vibrating energy—or patterns of activity—which are interconnected but are never seen, however, the effect of the dynamic patterns of energy can be measured. This concept can be related to a magnet. The energy field around the magnet cannot be seen, however, it can be felt when another magnet is near; it either attracts or repels the second magnet. So we can see the result of the dynamic energy as opposed to the dynamics of the energy itself. The arrangement of iron filings, can be seen, but not the force that produces the arrangement. The same is true of the wind and other natural phenomena.

Another quantum physics theory is that the energy in nature is not absorbed or radiated continuously. It is not a smooth and continuous flow but has gaps—silent gaps. These silent gaps are the home of the dynamic force of unexpressed form. The discoverer of these silent gaps, Max Planck called the phenomena quanta. The second advancement in thought was provided by Einstein's Theory of Relativity, $E=MC^2$. Einstein demonstrated to the scientific world a new relationship between energy, matter, gravity and light. His equation proved that matter can be converted into energy and thus unified matter is energy. Atoms become transformed energy.

The theory of relativity also gave a whole new concept of time. Our usual concept of time is linear. However, traveling at or near the speed of light time contracts, and depending on the observer, distance contracts. In quantum mechanics time fluctuates. The relativity of the sense of time was explained by Einstein very simply when he said, "If you sit with a beautiful girl, two hours seems like two minutes. If you sit on a hot stove, a few minutes seems like two hours. That is relativity." Relativity is linked with perceptions. So too is your health. If you perceive you are ill, you will become ill. The practitioner can assist in changing the perception by having a strong belief in the effectiveness of the therapy applied.

The fact that a person is alive and breathing, is an indication of a certain amount of energetic forces at work. Energy is necessary to get up and walk around and do things. Energy is the actual movement of body parts which creates and transforms energy producing heat and the regulation of body temperature. As the systems of the body work with and between each other to maintain our body as a whole, this requires an energy that cannot be seen. Again, the effects, whether it is conscious movement or unconscious movement via the autonomic nervous system, the creation of an idea, or the expression of feelings, all are proof of the manifestation of energy.

Like fingerprints everything down to each individual cell has its own unique frequency of energy or vibration—whether it can be weighed, seen, or measured. It is entirely possible that the science of today has yet to build sophisticated enough measuring devices to detect and measure all the different frequencies of energy. Until the work of the physicists in this century pushed the frontiers of physics further into a blending of material and non-material it was thought that the atom was the smallest unit of measurement. Now it is recognized that beyond the neutrons, electrons and protons of the atom are building blocks of hadrons called quarks and gluons. Though none of these have ever been seen, because of their energy, they are known to exist. In addition, each type of quark is thought to have three possible colors. Although the colors are called red, green, and blue, they are not related to visual colors.

Einstein acknowledged the knowledge of man was in its infancy. Further investigation of this brief discussion of quantum physics and energy could expand our consciousness about the role energy plays in our lives and specifically in healing. In addition, there are other forms of energy we must also consider.

Physiological Energy

About 300 years ago medicine made a decision to explain the body and work from a base founded on chemistry. That decision was understandable because chemistry was the most advanced science at the time and was the most rapid way for medicine to advance. In addition, medicine was primarily looking at the causes of disease.

Physiologically all activities of the body require energy, and all needs are met by the consumption of food containing energy in chemical form. The human diet comprises three main sources of energy: carbohydrates, proteins, and fats. Of these three, carbohydrates most readily provide the kind of energy needed to activate muscles while proteins work to build and restore body tissues. The body transforms chemical energy derived from food in the process called metabolism, an activity that takes place in the individual cells. Molecules of the food substances providing energy pass through the cell wall. Inside the cell, chemical reactions occur that produce new forms of energy and yield by-products such as water and waste materials.

To understand the body through chemistry again provides a singular dimensional view. In the past these singular views were investigated in order to gain an understanding of the body's function and structure. This led to a mechanical interpretation that was more consistent with Newtonian physics. As with physics, when one comes to the end of chemistry and its building blocks, we know there is something beyond it. Valerie Hunt, research scientist and healer, says research is proving that at the extreme end of chemistry is an electrical charge. When life starts there is an electromagnetic spark that activates chemistry. When we die, electromagnetic energy leaves the body. In essence, life is electromagnetic, not chemical. Today, electromagnetism can be measured, and Hunt feels, it is inevitable that a medicine based on this concept will become recognized. Fitzgerald, according to Ingham, concurred with this concept. She writes in 1945, "His [Fitzgerald's] theoretical explanation of results obtained is that the human body is an electro-mechanism."[3]

Biomechanics

There are many different kinds of energy at work in the body. Researchers who study the dynamics of walking feel human locomotion is largely a matter of transferring energy from one form to another. Shifting potential energy that is stored in flexible body tissues to kinetic energy produced by motion as the body takes a step. Yet, it appears the body does not lose any energy in this transference. In the 1949 classic, *Functional Foot Disorders,* Dr. John Martin Hiss reports on a study that discusses the kinetic energy used in walking. He writes, "An exacting study of the dynamics of human walking, by Elftman, has shown that a person walking on a level, at a constant average velocity, has done no work on the body in a physical sense, since he finishes with the same potential and kinetic energy as he had when he started."[4] We shall again look at this use of energy in more detail later in the chapter on biomechanics, but suffice it to say for now that the use of energy is a phenomena in walking and every step you take could be adversely affecting your body.

Mental Energy

Medically speaking, *nervous energy* is defined as constitutional vigor or strength. It is the term often associated with psychology. In the same vein, the term *psychic energy* or force is used in psychoanalysis to define a mental force regarded as corresponding in some respects to the physical concept of energy; in this case it is energy enabling and vitalizing an individual's psychological activity. Libido is defined as energy, motive force, desire or striving, either as derived from the sex instinct or from the primal urge to live.[5]

Historically, in 1913, Russian psychologist, Dr. Valdimir Bekhterev, coined the term reflexology, using it in discussing his doctrine of the study of the human personality. He comes very close to an energy concept when he speaks of the personality as being a manifestation of feeling, knowing, and willing or "the phenomena of psychic activity—the spiritual sphere."[6]

Today, psychic energy has to do with our mind and emotions which are beyond the known physical processes. Understanding how an emotion may be transformed into a physical illness requires knowledge of the mental process Freud called 'conversion'. He felt mental processes are characterized by energy and activity just as are the physical processes. The difference is that the activity of energy and mental processes cannot be seen, but the results are felt.

Writing in *Your Mind Can Cure*, Anita Stevens, M.D. (1974) says, "Thoughts never vanish. No thought is ever lost to the unconscious, which stores it forever. Charles Sherrington, Nobel Prize winner in physiology, showed that...the energy of the inhibited reflex did not disappear but persisted in undiminished strength, waiting to take effect later."[7] Stevens, a psychiatrist, goes on to write, [When we repress some action]...The natural discharge of

44

psychic energy attached to that wish-action is blocked. Then what happens? The energy of the psychic wish must find some discharge in order to restore 'constancy' to the mental processes of the mind. One way is through physical illness."[8]

According to Stevens, illness can provide the individual with an opportunity to reflect, in a non-judgmental way, and change his motives, or outlook on situations, and eventually his actions and reactions. Reflection is not based on a judgmental, simplistic rationale (e.g. your foot hurts so you are afraid of stepping forward). It requires time and most of all must be understood as a process. Through the exercise of reflection, comes an inner balance, an understanding of our true nature and approach to the world. Difficult circumstances often create attitudinal shifts, whole new frames of reference by which people see the world and themselves and others in it, and what life is asking of them. Illness or injury may be seen as a blessing in that it creates for us the time to slow down and to examine an unconscious dilemma or problem that requires our attention.

Energy Medicine

In *Vibrational Medicine*, Dr. Richard Gerber (1988) explains conventional medicine's use of energy today when he writes, "Orthodox medicine has begun to gradually explore the uses of energy for treating illness: Radiation to treat cancer, or electricity to alleviate pain and shrink tumors, electromagnetic fields to stimulate fracture healing and magnetic fields to alle-

viate the pain and inflammation of arthritis."[9] Perhaps in the not to distant future other forms of energy will be explored for their potential in healing.

Subtle Energies

Certain other 'subtle' energies are also known to exist and may produce the same healing processes. This energy comes from within and leads us into the distinction of energy levels. Gross energy levels are currently those that can be weighed, seen, and measured. While subtle energy levels are known to exist, the scientific technology to measure them is often lacking. Science has many times proven that subtle energies such as ultrasonics and microwaves can cause sickness, why cannot other subtle energies produce health? If it is true that the color of quarks are not related to visual colors, is it not possible there is an entire range of energy vibrations which manifests itself as colors that cannot be measured? Why is it that many people only believe what can be seen, weighed, or measured, when even science isn't that restrictive? Science admits there is a range of sound not heard by humans, and knows of a range of colors not perceived by sight. In so admitting, science moves out of the Newtonian machine model into a broader prospective of matter as energy.

In reality the building blocks of all life are particles of energy joining together to form physical matter. We are all the same energy, coalesced in different ways to create different forms and different matter. It is simply the same energy behaving differently.

As the subject of energy forms part of the philosophy of reflexognosy, it is an examination of this broader perspective of 'energy' to which we will now turn.

---

[1] Rossi, Laurence and David Cheek. *Mind-Body Therapy*, WW Norton, New York, 1994, pg xix.

[2] Stedman, Thomas. *Illustrated Stedman's Medical Dictionary*, Wilkins & Wilkins, Baltimore, 1982, pg. 466.

[3] Ingham, Eunice. *Zone Therapy It's Application to the Glands and Kindred Ailments*, 1945, pg. 5.

[4] Hiss, John Martin. *Functional Foot Disorders*, The Oxford Press, 1949, pg. 91.

[5] *Merriam-Webster New Collegiate Dictionary*, 1986, pg. 484.

[6] Bekhterev, Valdimir. *General principles of Human Reflexology*, International Publishers, New York, 1932, pg. 33.

[7] Stevens, Anita. *Your Mind Can Cure*, 1974, pg. 11.

[8] Stevens, pg. 13-14.

[9] Gerber, Richard. *Vibrational Medicine*, Bear & Company, Santa Fe NM, 1988, pg. 116.

Chapter 5

Subtle Energies & Energy Medicine

"Energy cannot be seen and understood except through its material manifestations."
—Chinese philosopher Nei Ching Ling Shu, two thousand years ago

This new model based on energy, has been embraced by people in the complementary field whose version of reality places importance on the unseen, and in the case of the human body, to human consciousness and the body/mind connection or the relatedness of the parts of the body to the whole organism.

The continual changes of one's organism in relation to the changing external environment will naturally include temporary phases of ill health, and it will often be impossible to draw a sharp line between health and illness, as health is really a multidimensional phenomenon involving interdependent physical, psychological and social aspects. The common acceptance of health and illness as opposite ends of a one-dimensional continuum is misleading. First, the system will adjust to stress. Second, physical disease may be balanced by a positive mental attitude and social support, so that the overall state is one of well-being. On the other hand, emotional problems or social isolation can make a person feel sick in spite of physical health.

Relating this concept of energy and wholism to the human body, we come to some fundamental beliefs upon which six medical systems are based. While they are all considered complementary medicine techniques or theories, the six energy medical models include:

Models of Energy Medicine

- **CHINESE TRADITIONAL MEDICINE**
  Chi
- **AYURVEDIC MEDICINE**
  Prana
- **HOMEOPATHIC MEDICINE**
  Vital Force
- **CHIROPRACTIC MEDICINE**
  Universal Consciousness
- **ANTHROPOSOPHICAL MEDICINE**
  Etheric/Life Force
- **HERBAL MEDICINE**
  Vital Force
  (or the chemical interchange with the vital force)

In these models all refer in some sense to the body's innate intelligence with the human body. Likened to a landscape embodying the five forces of nature—wood, fire, earth, metal, and water—this can be illustrated in a body like a garden with all kinds of analogies:

The Body as a Garden

- **Fire/air (mind/thoughts/emotions)**
- **Water/rivers (circulation/lymph;**
- **Earth/mountain (tissue/organs/glands)**
- **Wood/trees (spine/bones)**
- **Metal/chemical processes of the body (nutrition/digestion)**

Before proceeding, a few definitions are warranted so that we can view what follows from the same perspective. In checking *Webster's New World Dictionary* (1988) we find:

Holism is the view that an organic or integrated whole has an independent reality which cannot be understood through an understanding of its parts.[1] *Wholistic* as an adjective means to be concerned with, or dealing with wholes or integrated systems rather than their parts, e.g. wholistic health, dealing with the whole organism which includes the mind or body-mind connection. Reflexognosy is included in wholistic therapies with their emphasis in this direction.

The *brain* is a mass of tissue that is the main part of the nervous system. It is understood as being the center of thought and the organ that perceives sensory impulses and regulates motor impulses. The *mind* on the other hand is defined as the seat or subject of consciousness; the conscious and unconscious together as a unit. The use of the word unconscious in not meant in the conventional psychological term, but as an automatic working of the body that we are not directing by conscious thought. On one level the unconscious is the body's innate intelligence which 'thinks'. The body's innate intelligence or mind is in every cell of our bodies. Our conscious actions and thoughts combined by those performed unconsciously by the body's innate intelligence through the different systems of the body, i.e. digestion, communication via the nervous system, heart beating, blood circulation, etc. all contribute to the state of our being.

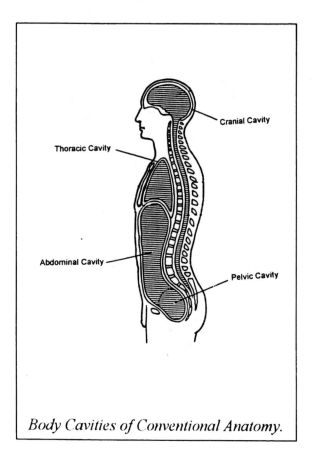

Body Cavities of Conventional Anatomy.

Illness is a condition of the total human being, *disease* is a condition of a particular part of the body.

A science concerned only with quantity and based exclusively on measurement is inherently unable to deal with experience, quality, or values. Since the human being is basically a dynamic process and health is harmony of this movement, this brings up an interesting concept about the division of the body into systems such as the nervous system, endocrine system, digestive system, etc. This division may soon be outmoded for everything is interconnected and each system relies on the others to function. The preceding illustration shows the conventional division of the body into four body cavities.

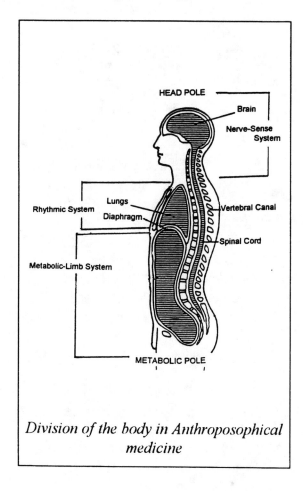

HEAD POLE

Brain

Nerve-Sense System

Rhythmic System

Lungs

Diaphragm

Vertebral Canal

Spinal Cord

Metabolic-Limb System

METABOLIC POLE

Division of the body in Anthroposophical medicine

Anthroposophical Medicine[2]

In Anthroposophical medicine, of which we will speak in more detail later, the body is divided into three cavities through a revolutionary way of viewing function. This in turn provides the theory that the maintenance of health is a matter of keeping the energies of the upper and lower poles of the body in balance. The upper pole of the body is represented by the nerve-sense system involving the head, where most of the sense organs are to be found, the brain and the spinal cord—the thinking part of our nature. The lower pole is called the metabolic-limb system involving the stomach, intestines—the movement of energy in the form of food/metabolism, and the limbs which move the entire body and are involved with the *will* part of our nature.

These two poles meet where the blood stream and the lungs come together in what is called the *rhythmic* system. The important word here is rhythm. Our pulse has a certain rhythm as does our breathing—both originating in the thoracic cavity. The rhythmic system includes the heart and lungs with the center of the activity in the solar plexus. As is well known, relaxation of the solar plexus is important for relaxation of the entire body. According to Ayurvedic medicine, achieving relaxation is the first step to healing. Because of the deep state of relaxation clients feel, we can say reflexognosy works in the rhythmic system bringing about a balance between the nerve-sense system and the metabolic-limb system, in turn, a balance in our thinking, feeling, and willing or in other words, a balancing of the connection between the body, mind, and spirit. In Chinese Medicine this balance is succinctly expressed as the balance of yin and yang. It appears the division of the body into cavities in both views is correct but different depending on the starting point. Both are useful, but one without the other is not wholistic. What is needed as we move into the 21st century is a blend of anatomy and physiology with energy concepts in order to address the multi-faceted and multi-dimensional individual.

Room does not allow an inclusive investigation of all the various forms of energy medicines, nor an in-depth discussion of those included in the coming section. The systems mentioned serve only as an example for reflexognosists to consider and ponder as reflexognosy focuses on all systems of the body, including the subtle energy systems, and does not view parts of the body in isolation, nor the physical body isolated from the mind, soul or spirit. The reader is encouraged to take courses and read books on the various disciplines mentioned to gain a clearer understanding of each tradition.

Vibrations

It is recognized that for anything to exist at all a certain level of energy is required. Whatever the form, all changes in energy give off a certain amount of heat. This change in energy can oftentimes be measured by degrees of heat shown through thermography and the action or the vibration it produces. When we speak of vibration, we are merely using another word to express the the rate of the movement of energy. Different

frequencies of energy reflect varying rates of vibration. We know that matter and energy are two different manifestations of the same primary energetic substance of which everything in the universe is composed, including our physical and subtle bodies, but recall science does not know precisely what energy is. The vibratory rate of this universal energy determines the density of its expression as matter. Matter which vibrates at a very slow frequency is referred to as physical matter. That which vibrates at speeds exceeding light velocity is known as subtle matter. The word vibrant is often used to describe the state of good health. This implies the balancing—the moving back and forth—of body energies to maintain health. The use of the term 'vibration' or 'vibratory' in relation to health is not new. It is one of the principles of homeopathy.

Homeopathy

In 1779 Samuel Hahnemann earned a conventional medical degree in Germany. But by 1792 he had become disenchanted with the medical practices of the day. From his own investigative research, partly by intuition and partly by logical reasoning, he found that substances which produced symptoms in a healthy person could remove similar symptoms in someone unhealthy. This became known as the law of similars, *similia similibus curentur*, select the remedy which produces a similar clinical picture.

A second law of homeopathy was uncovered as Hahnemann developed his remedies. Hahnemann experimented with various potencies because many medicinal ingredients were highly toxic. When he diluted them their curative powers were also reduced. However, he stumbled onto the concept of diluting the substance in water or alcohol and then shaking the bottle. The whole process of alternately diluting and shaking is known as the process of potentization. Hahnemann found that potentization, to the point that chemical analysis could not detect any material substance of the original substance, freed the remedy from toxicity and increased its curative powers. The vigorous process of potentization acts as a catalyst, releasing the inner vital energy of the substances.

Homeopathy is the development of chemistry at the etheric or subtle energy level. The way matter is potentized allows for the coding of molecules through the intention of the person mixing the matter and the subtle energy of the substance. Homeopathy deals with the law of similars. Reflexognosy also deals with the law of similars in regard to the shape of the body being replicated on the foot. This concept was discussed more fully in Chapter Two.

Chiropractic and Universal Consciousness

Chiropractic has a long history dating back to ancient times in various regions of the world before the time of Christ. Modern chiropractic traces its roots to D. D. Palmer when, in 1895 as a healer, he accidentally aligned a vertebrae that was not in its normal position. This adjustment healed the client's deafness instantaneously. In 1897 Palmer opened the first Chiropractic school in Davenport, Iowa. The philosophy, science, and art of chiropractic is dedicated to restoring normal nerve transmission in the body and further, to maintaining that normality through the proper alignment of the spine. It is based on the premise that every system and each organ within each system is coordinated and regulated by the master controlling system of the brain and spinal cord. When the vertebrae of the spine become misaligned (subluxed) the resulting pressure interferes with the transmission of nerve impulses from the brain to organs and other tissues of the body. Left unattended the subluxation over a period of time may result in pain and disease.

Chiropractic adjustments have become greatly refined over the years. Today, going back to D.D. Palmer's belief in the body's ability to heal itself through its innate intelligence, a growing group of chiropractors, calling their work Network Chiropractic, deal with releasing and energizing the life force of the body. Their concern is with the nervous system's role in the free communication between the brain and spinal cord *and* the emotional, mental, and physical aspects of the body.

According to their philosophy, it is the life force which heals. The energy or life force is channeled through the nervous system and directed by a 'Universal Consciousness' or the body's innate intelligence. This intelligence is that part of the body that animates, motivates, coordinates, and inspires us to heal and repair. It is that source of knowledge that knows to tell the heart to beat and the lungs to breathe. The activities which happen without a person consciously thinking and willing them to happen. Subluxations interfere with the body's ability to

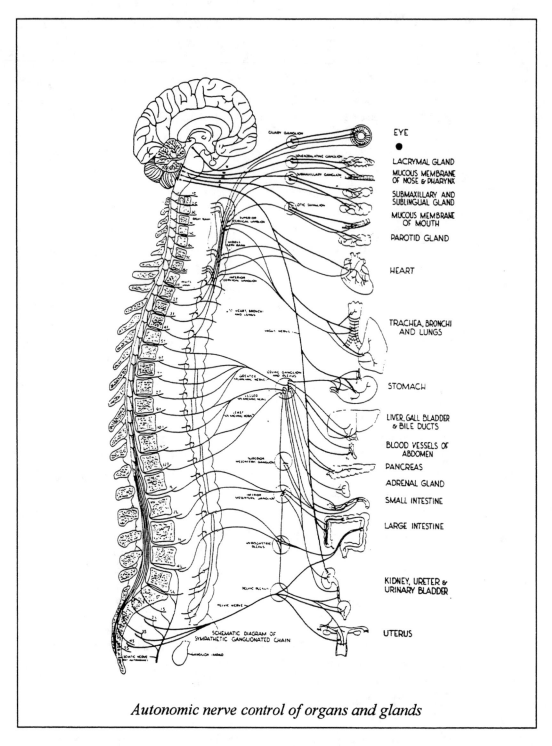

Autonomic nerve control of organs and glands

carry out the commands of it's innate intelligence.

While the focus in chiropractic is the spine, The complementary use of reflexognosy in this regard is dynamic, due to the influence the feet and legs have on 'balance' and moving anatomy. Structural deviations from normalcy in the foot will create imbalances which will affect every part of the body, either directly, or indirectly. Indirectly there will be an influence on the autonomic nerve ganglia and hence to the organs and glands.

Chinese Traditional Medicine and Chi

Williams (1995) writes, "it should be remembered that Chinese medicine operates very much at a subtle energy level. Qi, Blood, Jing and Shen are essentially energetic properties that continually oscillate around the cusp of the physical and the energetic."[3]

In Traditional Chinese Medicine, which is the most widely used healing system in the world, the body is viewed from a different perspective than conventional western medicine and has resulted in different thoughts and beliefs. As Ted Kaptchuk so succinctly says, "In Chinese medicine, as in Chinese philosophy, one cannot understand the whole until one knows parts and cannot understand the parts without knowing the whole."[4]

Their idea of striving for the balance of energy [chi] uses a different vocabulary to describe what they consider the dynamic energy of the body. Because of cultural restraints rather than the development and use of the vocabulary of Western science they have used the vocabulary of the poet. Chinese Traditional Medicine strives to balance chi using a variety of techniques including acupuncture, moxibustion, acupressure, massage, and herbs.

The classical acupuncture theory believes that life energy flows through the body along a series of pathways known as meridians. Meridians is an English word taken from geography that indicates an imagined line connecting a series of points. The meridians reflect imbalances in the energy system and then act as channels by which the imbalance can be corrected. Along the twelve meridians are specific points which sit just under the skin and conduct energy. Acupuncture is a two-way communication between the skin and all the organs and glands and tissue of the body. Each meridian is said to be associated with a particular organ, hence their names. When one or more meridians become blocked, the energy stagnates and disease results. By touching certain points on the skin, the energy flow is stimulated or sedated. Acupuncture seeks to remove the blocks and help restore the internal energy balance the body requires to heal itself. While acupuncture manipulates areas with the use of fine needles placed in a variety of locations, these same points may be stimulated or sedated by direct pressure in acupressure until proper energy flow is restored. Other things besides needles and pressure are also utilizied to balance chi. For instance, moxibustion uses the smoldering tinder [moxa] of the mugwort herb to stimulate energy sites along the body.

Dr. Richard Gerber, (1988) in his book *Vibrational Medicine* cites the work of a team of Korean researchers in the 1960s headed by Professor Kim Bong Han which focused their experimental work on the acupuncture meridians of animals. "Based on many experiments, Kim concluded that the meridian system not only inter-linked within itself but appeared to interconnect with all cell nuclei of the tissues."[5] Kim confirmed the importance of continuous meridian flow to particular organs via the deep meridian systems. Reports Gerber, "He [Kim] severed the meridian going to the liver in a frog and studied subsequent microscopic changes in the liver tissue. Shortly after severing the liver meridian, the hepato-cytes enlarged and their cytoplasm became very turbid. Within three days, serious vascular degeneration took place throughout the whole liver."[6] In addition, "Kim discovered that the formation of the acupuncture meridian system preceded the development and placement of rudimentary organs in the embryo. His work suggests that some type of information flows through the meridians to the DNA control centers of the cells, providing additional modulation to the embryologic developmental process."[7]

Acupuncture Meridians

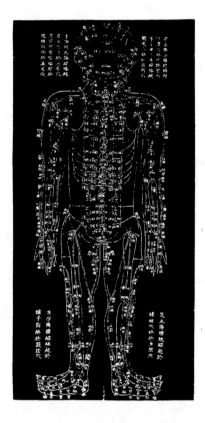

All of the meridians can be found in the feet. While reflexognosists do not directly work with acupuncture points they do stimulate the points indirectly while working on the tissue of the feet.

There are external and internal meridians. Internal meridians are too deep to be reached directly and go to major organs. External meridians can be reached through acupuncture needles and pressure. Meridians are a warning system. The acupuncture meridian system is a discretely organized network of microscopic ducts which connect the physical to the subtle energy etheric body, forming the so-called physical/etheric interface.

It is interesting to note from a historical perspective, that according to Richard Grossman, M.D. (1985) in his book *The Other Medicines*, acupuncture was actually known in America over one hundred years ago. He writes, "A doctor in South Carolina, for instance, reported in the *Boston Medical and Surgical Journal*, of September 14, 1836, that 'acupuncture owes its efficacy to the transmission of galvanic fluid.... It is not inconvenient. Every house can furnish needles, It is prompt and effectual. I have never failed to produce the desired effect, in appropriate cases, within the space of a quarter of an hour; and in such cases the relief was permanent.'"[8]

Acupuncture has grown in acceptance among the scientific community as a direct result of research linking acupuncture analgesia with the release of endorphins within the central nervous system. The endorphin model gave scientific theorists the first conclusive experimental evidence for acupunture's link with known pain pathways in the brain and spinal cord.

In a study with human subjects, using fMRI image equipment, Korean physicist Zang-Hee Cho at the University of California, Irvine [a non-believer of acupuncture] conducted an experiment contrasting response by the brain to stimulation of the eye by a light flashed in front of the subject versus manipulation of acupoints on the lateral side of the foot. The points stimulated run from the small toe to the ankle [BL67, BL66, BL65, and BL60] on the bladder meridian. These point are traditionally used to treat visions problems. Much to Cho's surprise, as reported in Discover magazine, "he found sticking a needle into someone's foot had the very same effect as shining a light in someone's eyes. And this was not the generalized analgesic effect, produced by the primitive limbic system, that was seen in the pain studies; this was a function-specific response occurring in the brain's cortex." Up until this time it was thought by acupuncture proponents that there was little connection between the brain and various organs and that stimulating an acupoint sent a message to the targeted organ directly and did not go through the brain. "Moreover," the article continues, "the magnitude of brain activity seen on acupuncture stimulation was nearly as strong as that elicited by the flash of light."

"To eliminate the possibility of a placebo effect, Cho also stimulated a nonacupoint, in the big toe. There was no response in the visual cortex."

Cho also noticed something else of interest. "When the activation data were graphed to show the intensity of the response over time, he saw that there were two distinct reactions among the dozen volunteers. During the acupuncture phase, some showed an increase in activity, while others showed a decrease. In other words,

in some people, oxygen consumption in the brain region increased, while in others it decreased." This was attributed, by an acupuncturist, to the balancing of yin and yang. [9]

No mention of the meridians would be complete without a few words about the five elements [fire, wood, earth, water, and metal] of Chinese Medicine which are concerned with function of the various structures in the body. Each of the elements is associated with specific parts of the body. Furthermore, to the Chinese an organ is considered more than its structure. It more closely corresponds to what we in the West would consider a system of the body. For instance, the organ of the heart includes the heart, the blood vessels, the energy of the blood circulation, as well as the blood tissue. When a practitioner speaks in terms of a 'liver problem' that is not to say there is necessarily a problem with the function of the physical liver, but the blockage or disturbance is within the liver meridian and all the seen and unseen elements that compose or are influenced by that meridian.

The elements are also related to a season of the year, climate, orifice, sense organ, body part/tissue, fluid secretion, physical manifestation, emotion, sound, flavor, and color.

The unique nature of the meridians is to reflect imbalance and then to act as the channel by which the imbalance can be corrected. 'Treatment is diagnosis and diagnosis is treatment'. Reflexognosists influence major meridians housed in the feet and legs by their carefully selected techniques. They blend stimulating and sedating techniques as warranted by the client presentation.

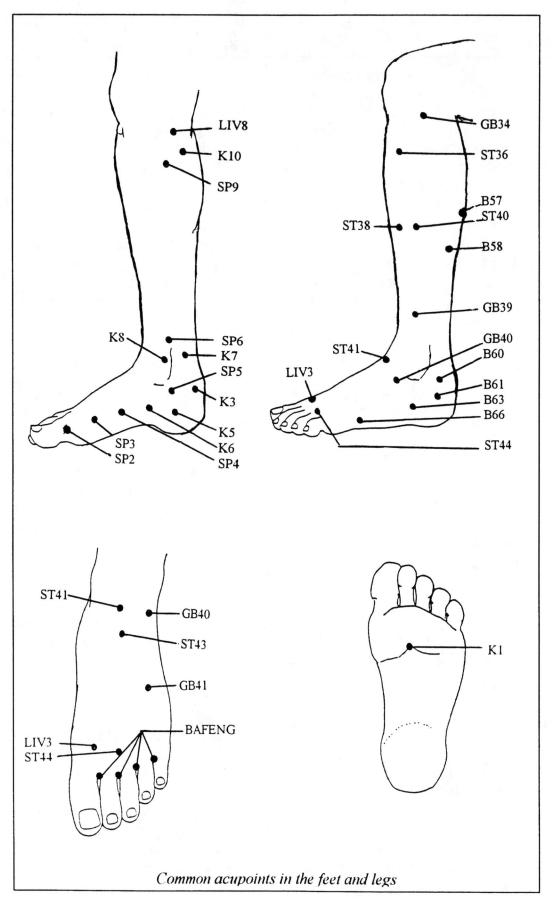

Common acupoints in the feet and legs

Meridians and the general principals associated with this field of health care must be considered as one major reason why such profound results are achieved with reflexognosy.

Ayurvedic Medicine and Prana

Ayurvedic medicine (*Ayur*: health and *Veda*: teaching), means the science of long life. It is another ancient system of healing based on folk wisdom and energy. Ayurvedic medicine has a 5,000 year history in India. It is wholistic in concept and incorporates the entire body based on preventive medicine and harmony and balance from within. Ayurvedic medicine defines the physical world in terms of energy—*prana*—which is actually a moving stream of particles that can be arranged and rearranged at will. Disease is defined as a state of mind in which your energy is out of the order in which it normally flows. The mind is a key to health and influences the body. There are subdivisions within this science. An Ayurvedic doctor will type and match the way he believes your mind and body speak to one another. Generally a person is one of three predominating mind/body types or *dosha*. The *pitta* is intense and critical, the *vata* is changeable and excitable, and the *kapha* dosha is relaxed and forgiving. Once an illness is diagnosed, specific foods, herbs, massage techniques, exercises or aromas are prescribed to balance the energy.

Ayurvedic medicine divides the body into ten zones. Each zone corresponds to the five elements from which all life is formed: ether, air, fire, water, and earth similar to the elements in Chinese Medicine. The

The Five Elements	
Ayurveda	Chinese
Ether	Wood
Air	Metal
Fire	Fire
Water	Water
Earth	Earth

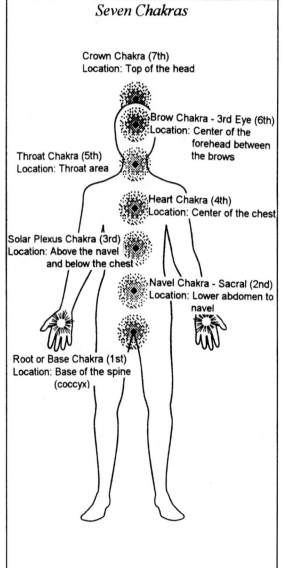

Seven Chakras

Crown Chakra (7th)
Location: Top of the head

Brow Chakra - 3rd Eye (6th)
Location: Center of the forehead between the brows

Throat Chakra (5th)
Location: Throat area

Heart Chakra (4th)
Location: Center of the chest

Solar Plexus Chakra (3rd)
Location: Above the navel and below the chest

Navel Chakra - Sacral (2nd)
Location: Lower abdomen to navel

Root or Base Chakra (1st)
Location: Base of the spine (coccyx)

Location of the seven major chakras or energy centers. There are also powerful energy centers in the palms of the hands and the soles of the feet.

traditional 'elements were symbols for certain energic [energy] forces or tendencies...aspects of nature and of our bodymind nature."[10] The zones in Ayurveda are the channels through which the *chakras* direct the flow of prana through the body, just as major arteries carry blood from the heart for distribution to all cells. According to Deepak Chopra (1991), gently working the backs of the ears is especially good for quieting the excitable personality.[11] This is the dosha responsible for all movement of the body and one of the three basic metabolic principles connecting the mind and body.

Chakras

In acupuncture the energy flows through meridians which correspond to the organs, the circulation and lymph systems. In Ayurvedic medicine energy flows through *chakras* which correspond to the glands, the nervous, and endocrine systems. The chakras are specialized energy centers in the subtle bodies, each associated with a major nerve and glandular center in the physical body. The endocrine glands effect the body from a cellular level up to the functioning of the central nervous system. The chakras are thus able to affect our moods and behavior through hormonal influences on brain activity.

The chakras are connected to each other and to various aspects of the physical body through energetic threads known as nadis, together forming the chakra-nadi network. The chakra-nadi system connects the organic/molecular form with the organizational energies of the etheric body.

Each of the seven major cha-kras has particular glands and organs, functions, color, and elements associated with it. Also certain physical, emotional, and spiritual issues affect a chakra's proper functioning. When an individual has significant unresolved issues in any one of these areas, chakra dysfunction may occur. Such dysfunction leads to deprivation of nutritive subtle-energy flow to the bodily region and associated organs and glands supplied by the impaired chakra. If the chakra blockage is chronic, cellular imbalance and disease will eventually occur.

As with reflexes, it is very easy to fall into the trap of simplistic thinking—focusing on a particular chakra for a certain dysfunction rather than studying the chakras in depth then supporting and balancing the entire subtle energy of the body. For this reason the authors avoid giving the specifics here and encourage the reader to study the chakras in greater detail.

Anthroposophical Medicine

Anthroposophical Medicine, of which much has already been referred, stems from the inspiration of Austrian mystic Rudolf Steiner (1865-1925). Training in Anthroposophical Medicine is open only to those already educated as conventional medical doctors and then further their studies medically by delving into the spiritual workings of the body as viewed from Anthroposophy or Spiritual Science. In Anthroposophical medicine, the maintenance of health is viewed as a matter of keeping the energies of the upper and lower poles of the body in balance as well as balancing the connection between body, mind, and spirit in connection with the person's destiny.

Vitalogy and Vital force

In closing this discussion on subtle energy healing systems the vitalogists must also be mentioned. Toward the end of the 19th century and leading into the early part of the 20th century there was a respected group of healers called vitalogists. They adhered to the doctrine that the life in living organisms is caused and sustained by a vital force that is distinct from all physical and chemical forces. The physio-medical philosophy was that the physical basis of life was vital not chemical. Today this vital force is known as the electromagnetic field.

The history of vitalogy or the use of herbs in medicine has been handed down to the present day medical herbalists in the West and Chinese herbalists in the East. Western history begins with Hippocrates. This tradition was kept alive in the 1600s by the work of Dr. William Fox, in the 1700s with Samuel Thompson, and in the 1890s with Dr. T.J. Lyle. Lyle was a professor of therapeutics and materia medica in Chicago at the Physio Medical College.

Professor Lyle also held to the idea that energy imbalance, either in excess or insufficiency was the root of all illness. "Altered physiology" a termed coined by him is the state where the body moves away from internal harmony. He did not identify altered physiology with specific disease names. Instead the aim of the practitioner is to restore the 'vital force'.

In conjunction with restoring vital force, the healing properties (chemistry) and life force within plants or herbs are employed in place of the chemicals of conventional medicine. The isolation of some specific therapeutic principles from a plant has proved to be a good remedy, but long experience has taught that, by keeping these therapeutic or 'active' principles in context, or 'organized', in the whole plant, the patient is less likely to suffer the side effects now so common in modern drug therapy. The use by the herbalist of the whole plant rather than an extract, such as an alkaloid used in isolation, is the very important difference between the traditional herbalist and the allopathic doctor today. Herbalists believe that the removal, or isolation, of a therapeutic principle from the many other vital constituents in the rest of the plant, known or unknown, detracts from the healing ability of the product.

Vitality of the Foot

Dr. John Martin Hiss (1949) uses the term *vitality* in reference to the life process that permeates the foot as it does other body tissues. Vitality he defines as life itself and divides the process of vitality into four parts:

1. Intelligence—the mind

2. Switchboard control—the nervous system

3. Maintenance—the food supply

4. Circulation—or waste elimination.

Intelligence is the mind, spirit, soul, or deity according to one's viewpoint. "Intelligence is the life current that comes from an unknown origin, flows out through the nerve trunks and vitalizes cells to perform their functions. Neurologists have attempted to explain function on a basis of reactions to stimuli, reactions to environment, et cetera, but they are always confronted with the intelligence displayed in these reactions. Biochemists have explained a lot with their theories of colloids, and organic chemical reactions in tissues, but never have they understood the intelligence used by these cells in their selective functioning. Histologists and physiologists are confronted with the same unknown quantity when they describe protoplasmic structure and changes during cell activity."[12] "Intelligence," Hiss says, "is a state that no one seems to have intelligence enough to understand." He is convinced that it is not a physical thing, as evidenced by autopsies on the insane, which shows them to have "a physical brain equal to that of the most learned and talented of geniuses."[13]

Fascia

A close correlation can be drawn between vitality and fascia of the body. Fascia is soft tissue. It binds and supports the body but has recently been found to be the primary communication channel in the body. Fascia is a sheath that surrounds everything in the body, from the smallest nerve and muscle fiber to the largest bone, muscle and organ. Effective body work enhances tissue quality and thereby enhances the balance and flow of energy. It aids in speeding up the recovery of soft tissue by removal of dead cells, influencing venous and lympathic flow, thereby increasing the healing rate at which the body repairs itself physically. If there is a fascial restriction there is an energy restriction and vice versa. As palpation skills are developed the ability to feel these 'strain patterns' on a subtle energy level develop.

Subtle Energy Bodies

Energy can also be defined as strength of expression; force of utterance; life; spirit.[14] This definition contains within it a wholism. The concept of the body composed of numerous energetic forces which combines to form a whole organism is very important in the concept of health. Good health depends upon the maintenance of a harmonious balance between these different energetic forces and that all matter flows freely. There is only one disease: congestion. Congestion leads to stagnation.

In one sense we do not just take in energy; we are energy. The organs of our body are made of tissues made of cells, molecules, and atoms, which are all whirling, pulsating, vibrating fields of energy. Energy not only surrounds us it interpenetrates the cells of our body. All matter has vibration that, in turn, has a frequency. Within the body are different energy systems. On the gross or physical level [i.e., the physical level comprising the most dense level of energy] there are the biochemical and bioelectrical networks of the body. Then there are higher energies or a life-force responsible for life and creative expression. This network involves the work of the finer subtle energy systems of acupuncture meridians and the chakra-nadis.

The Tiller-Einstein Model

attempts to mathematically describe the behavior of energy/matter at velocities beyond the speed of light in order to establish a reality base for subtle energies and subtle bodies which are beyond ordinary human perception. According to the Tiller-Einstein model the first level of energies moving faster than light velocity are the etheric frequencies of matter and energy. Matter and energy are primarily electrical in nature. Matter is composed of particles such as the electron and proton, which are electrically charged. Whereas the energy/matter beyond the speed of light is electro*magnetic* in nature.

Life Force

Life-force is a subtle form of electromagnetic energy. It is the animating current of life and a physiological reality in the body. Through the centuries, life force has been called by different names. Among them are: 'bioplasmic energy' according to Russian psychic research, 'prana' by the East Indians, 'chi' by Chinese Traditional Medicine, Mesmer referred to it as 'magnetic fluid', and Hippocrates called it 'nature's life force'.

This life-force flows through the body as if it were following an invisible circulatory system, charging every cell in its path. This current of energy can become weakened or partially blocked due to stress. Acupuncture involves locating the exact points where blockage occurs and using needles, stimulates these points to restore flow. In polarity energy balancing, physical and nonphysical touch techniques are used to send energy through the entire system to open up the blocked points, re-establishing the proper flow and alignment of life-force throughout the body.

Electro-Magnetic Current

As strange as a life energy may sound, a new medical science of energy medicine is now emerging, in western culture thanks to the research of Dr. Robert Becker, (1985) a respected orthopedic surgeon and author of *The Body Electric* and *Cross Currents*. His experiments prove the body is more than a chemical and mechanical machine, it is also an electrical unit operating within an electrical web and an electrical energetic field surrounding the body. Research is showing that electromagnetic energy flows along pathways bearing some resemblance to meridians. Dr. Becker has documented the existence of an underlying electromagnetic life force within the body that stimulates it to grow and heal. His studies show that an injury causes the brain to send low-level electrical signals to the wound that stimulates repair. As the repair process continues this signal diminishes in intensity. The slower stimulating signal in turn slows the repair activity and when the wound heals the signal stops. Becker found if the current level is down in a very low range—around a pico amphere—one gets regeneration. If it is much higher than that one gets cell degeneration. This may explain the healing properties of relaxation, biofeedback, and meditation; all of which calm and slow the body down. It may also explain why some tactile therapists find slower movements constitute a stronger therapy which gives them access to the inner depths of the client both physically and emotionally.

In a lecture delivered in 1983, Dr. William Tiller shared that very low currents can modulate or balance the electromagnetics of current waves which is known as *magnetic vector potential*. Low currents, Tiller thinks, restores the vitality balance in organs by stimulating the body's magnetic vector potential. Tiller went on to postulate that slow acting low current processes subtle changes on the cellular level which can build up slowly and gradually produce significant changes over time.[15] This leaves us with the question: Is working slowly more advantageous than working fast, just as it may be more beneficial to use light to moderate pressure than heavy pressure?

Becker has also found that the points along the acupuncture meridians enhance the electromagnetic current flowing in the body. It was detected that the meridians had the electrical characteristics of transmission lines, while skin not associated with meridians did not. Electromagnetic medicine may be the science that unites both Eastern and Western philosophies in such a way that conventional medicine can come to appreciate what the methods beyond drugs and surgery have to offer and blend all into a new model.

Matter of different frequencies can coexist in the same space, just as energies of different frequencies of radio, cellular phones, and TV can exist nondestructively in the same space. The etheric and physical bodies forms of energy, being of different frequencies overlap and coexist within the same space.

The life-force or energy/matter of the anatomy of the subtle body, explains Richard Gerber,

(1988) seems to possess negative entropic* characteristics which in turn moves the cellular system toward the maintenance of balance instead of decay.[16] These negative entropic qualities are found in the fields of psychic healers. Anyone who has the ability to stimulate healing in others is able to provide an energetic boost to push the client's own energetic system back into balance where healing begins.

Although the digestive system takes in biochemical energy and molecular building blocks in the form of physical nutrients, the chakras, in conjunction with the acupuncture meridian system, take in higher vibrational energies that are just as integral to the proper growth and maintenance of physical life. Whereas the physical nutrients are used to promote cellular growth and homeostasis at the molecular level, the subtle-energy currents conveyed by the chakras and meridians assist in promoting stability and organization in the etheric body. The etheric body is the energy growth template for the physical. Energetic changes occur at the etheric level before becoming manifest as physical cellular events.

Placebo Effect

It is argued by some members of the scientific community that complementary therapies like reflexognosy work because of the placebo effect. While research has shown the

---

* Entropy is a term used to describe the state of disorder of a system. The greater the disorder the higher the entropy. Most processes in the physical world over time develop toward a higher entropy. Living organisms utilize energy to create balance within their physiologicial systems.

placebo effect is present within conventional drugs studies, science is more critical when the concept is applied to complementary therapies. However, often in chronic diseases the client has been previously treated with orthodox drugs, in which he or she had every confidence, with no benefit. Why then should the success of complementary therapies be dismissed as the placebo effect? It may mean that some intrinsic healing power, a blend of the subtle energies or influences, flows from or through the practitioner to the client which has nothing to do with whether or not the client believes in the therapy or the client's confidence in the practitioner. We shall have more to say about the placebo effect shortly when we discuss Franz Mesmer and his work.

Reflexognosy and Energy

Dr. Alfons Cornelius (1902) in his work, *Pressure Points, Their Origin and Significance* puts forth his hypothesis that the results he achieved with the application of pressure to points on the body followed the *vibratory* laws of acoustics. "One tone can in turn call forth another tone with the similar number of oscillations."[17] On the other hand, Cornelius felt the application of pressure worked within the nervous system in a purely mechanical way by hindering the neurons of the sympathetic nervous system. He indicated that the reaction to pressure raced through the body and triggered reactions far distant from the site where pressure was applied. This could lead one to question whether the vibratory reaction described by Cornelius was of a more

subtle nature, working on the electromagnetic energy field of the body.

In *Zone Therapy* Dr. William Fitzgerald and Edwin Bowers (1917) give the following four reasons for the way in which zone therapy works.[18]

1. "(through) the soothing influence of animal magnetism"

2. pressure over the injured place tends to prevent bruising

3. pressure over the injury blocks signals of injury to the brain

4. pressure can relieve pain and act as an anesthesia.

Two other theories are later given:

1. Following a relief in nerve tension, constriction or congestive conditions of the lymphatic glands or ducts, the thyroid and other ductless glands and vasomotor nerves occurs and is the reason for glandular and circulatory changes noted

2. Through the ultra-microscopic connections to nerves.

Returning to the discussion of subtle energy, the concept of animal magnetism as mentioned by Fitzgerald is most important. This concept was the work of Dr. Franz Mesmer. In the late 1700s Dr. Mesmer (1734-1815) claimed that the healing results he obtained came through the use of a vital force or universal energy, not through the patient's belief in him or through the patient's faith and belief in Jesus. It was not necessary for either the provider or the patient to fully understand or believe in the theory of energy manipulation in order for the techniques to be helpful. This broad view expressed by Fitzgerald confirms that the zones may have been only areas of reference.

In his early medical career Mesmer found that placing a magnet over areas of the body with a pathology would result in healing. To him this suggested that all things in nature—minerals, plants, animals and human beings—possessed a specific power or energy which he saw as a fluid. He believed that when an individual was in a state of health, he or she was in harmony with this basic law of nature.

He theorized that this subtle-life energy was magnetic, somehow associated with the nervous system, and was exchanged between healer and patient during the 'laying-on-of-hands'. Thus he termed laying-on-of-hands 'magnetic healing' or 'animal magnetism' The use of the word 'animal magnetism' had no sexual connotation at the time. It was used to distinguish this type of magnetism from the traditional magnetism of inorganic iron. Mesmer felt the most active points for this energy flow were found in the palms of the hands. Hence when the practitioner placed his hands on a patient, energy flowed from the healer to the patient. According to Richard Gerber (1988) "There are natural energy circuits involving the hands which take energy in through the left palm chakra and send energy out through the right."[19]

Professional life during Mesmer's time was not much different than today. Mesmer's colleagues credited his success to the placebo effect, or more accurately to hypnosis and the power of suggestion. In 1784 the King of France appointed members of the Academy of Sciences, the Academy of Medicine, the Royal Society, and Benjamin Franklin, to study Mesmer's work. Although they did not deny Mesmer's results, they concluded that the theory of a magnetic fluid did not exist. Nearly five decades later, in 1831, Mesmer's work was again investigated, this time by the Medical Section of the Academie des Sciencies, which overturned the previous opinion and accepted Mesmer's viewpoint. However, scientific damage had been done and Mesmer's work never achieved widespread recognition, even though he achieved exceptional results.

While direct measurement of these subtle energies by conventional tools today is difficult at best, recent laboratory investigations into the physiological effects of laying-on-of-hands are confirming the magnetic nature of subtle healing energies and that Mesmer's understanding of the magnetic energies of the body was somewhat correct.

Nearly one hundred years after Mesmer's death in 1815, Dr. Fitzgerald gives credit to animal magnetism as responsible for the results obtained with zone therapy. Fitzgerald must have felt zone therapy worked beyond the physical body and into other areas, whether it be by mental or other energy phenomena.

In turn, Fitzgerald surely found a willing pupil in Dr. Joe Shelby Riley of the theory of animal magnetism as he trained him in zone therapy. Riley was no stranger to alternative ways of thinking. He was a very open-minded physician. His practice of medicine was eclectic. He advertised that he practiced allopathic medicine and surgery, physiotherapy which included electrotherapy, thermo-therapy, zone therapy, spinal therapy which included chiropractic concussion, sinu soidalization and mechano-therapy, along with osteopathy and homeopathy.

Riley's background in chiropractic is noteworthy. Daniel David Palmer (1845-1913), the father of modern chiropractic believed the body, as did all living matter, possessed an 'innate intelligence' that was ultimately responsible for the very existence, survival, and growth of all living organisms. Palmer concluded the governing control mechanism for the innate intelligence was the nervous system. For a person to experience good health there must be an unobstructed flow of nerve impulses from the brain through the spinal nerves and out to every part of the body. Chiropractic manipulations relieve the blocks to spinal alignment thus maintaining health.*

In his book *Conquering Units: or the Mastery of Disease*, Shelby (1921) writes, "Chiropractic had its beginning in the year 1895, when the great old *magnetic* healer [a precursor to modern hypnotherapy],

---

* Out of chiropractic has come Dr. John Thie's *Touch for Health* which goes even further in working on what it calls the 'energy flow' in the human body. Touch for Health's approach to restoring our natural energies is by applying pressure, with the hands, on points associated with the structural and mechanical aspects of the body throughout the entire musculoskeletal system, not just the spine. Touch for Health combines many of the basic principles of Chinese medicine with chiropractic and brings chiropractic more into the field of energy medicine.

D.D. Palmer, succeeded in adjusting the 5th [thoracic] dorsal vertebra in the spine of one, Harvey Lilliard, a janitor of mixed blood, in the building where D.D. Palmer had his office. This was after treatment in magnetic healing had been continued for a long time without any results...."[20] This indicates that magnetic healing was an established form of healing, at least in America, when Fitzgerald was formulating zone therapy. [Emphasis and parenthesis added by Rogers & Issel.]

Riley was no stranger to 'mysticism' either. In 1959 Health Research compiled a 13 lesson course on numerology, or the vibration of numbers, written by Riley with another course, of again 13 lessons, by Mrs. L. Dow Balliett under the title *Numerology & Vibration*. "Numerology is the study of vibration. Everything in this world is moving or vibrating at a certain rate of speed. To simplify the study we say that thought waves—the power that compels our acts—is vibrating at a certain speed,"[21] writes Riley. This all sounds very much like electromagnetism.

Eunice Ingham (1951) spent a great deal of time writing about mental energy or vibrations in her work *Stories the Feet Have Told*. "We are constantly throwing out a certain amount and quality of vibration which shows the type of our personality."[22] She then goes on in the following twelve pages to discuss the effect of emotions on health and the mind/body connection. She was a remarkable pioneer, decades ahead of her time.

Reflexognosy and Subtle Energies

In the West the concept of the flow of chi, or the use of energy flow as a basis of understanding health or illness has not been acceptable. Now, thanks to modern science we are talking about invisible phenomenon or energy that no one sees yet believes to exist. The energy concept has been taken out of the realm of Oriental mysticism or 'New Age' hocus-pocus into that of quantum physics. This coupled with advancements in biology, chemistry, and electromagnetic research may bring about the blending of Eastern and Western concepts of energy.

Energy is a word which has many interpretations and assumes many forms. But it has been shown that on the physical level the concept is no stranger to Western science. Even the idea of energy is a concept. It is invisible. Only the results can be examined. Scientists have many times proven that subtle energies such as ultrasonic and microwaves can cause sickness. Why cannot other subtle energies produce health? It is the forms of energy which cause debate. While a practitioner of Chinese Traditional Medicine may alter the flow of chi in the body, a Western researcher, would describe it as changing the flow of direct current.

Reflexognosy draws together the Western scientific thoughts of quantum physics and reflex action with Eastern healing methods and philosophies to create a therapy of the future. From the Eastern philosophies we are stimulating by hand pressure many powerful acupuncture points in the feet along with the chakras. We are also stimulating meridians which distribute the vital energy

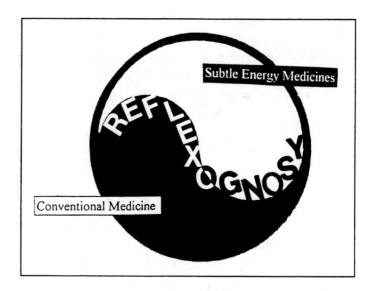

force through the body to bring a rich supply to feed our organs and mind.

It is important to consider that the master points of the six main meridians are found on the feet. Thus stimulating these meridians together with the physiological response via the circulatory, lymphatic and nervous systems validates the potency of reflexognosy.

Gaining knowledge of meridians, the five element theory, chakras and subtle energies of the etheric body can help reflexognosists understand the blockage of energy more comprehensively, and build a basic understanding of how their work can be of enormous benefit in balancing the body through influencing the meridians. However, it is not necessary to embrace Eastern mysticism or 'New Age' mysticism to work with energy. Though reflexognosists use models of chakras and meridians they translate this to anatomy and physiology because it allows the therapist to blend energy work with manual therapy so it does not trigger negative associations with clients or other health care providers. In the future, it may well be proven that reflexognosy is a bridge between traditional and vibrational medicine because it seemingly produces chemical and electrical changes in the body as well as changes in the electromagnetic fields.

Reflexognosy, due to its ability to assist in decongesting the body via stimulation to the circulatory, lymphatic, and nervous systems directly, would be a complementary therapy to consider for homeopaths. It does this with acupuncture also and works indirectly with the subtle energies housed within the meridians. Reflexognosy can correlate with Ayurvedic Medicine because of its effect on the glands of the endocrine system and the deep state of relaxation it usually produces. Reflexognosy assists the vital force of Vitalogy on several physical and energy planes. Distortions in the subtle anatomy may precede physical/cellular changes by some time. Beal (1980) points

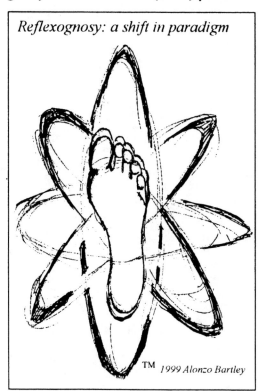

Reflexognosy: a shift in paradigm

TM *1999 Alonzo Bartley*

out that reflex activity may be noted before symptoms of visceral change

occur. When such changes become chronic, various tissue changes will be noted by the therapist. These signs, he notes, disappear if the viscera improves.[23] This may explain why a reflexognosist can detect a sensitive area on the foot before a pathological condition manifests. The correction of a potential disease or dysfunction is difficult to prove scientifically or medically because there is nothing left behind to indicate there was a potentially dangerous pre-existing condition.

Whether we are prepared to accept it or not it appears that health is a balance between our subtle energies and the gross energies of our physical body. Science and medicine are on the verge of a major shift based on the new research in energy and energy fields. For reflexognosists this means a blending of East and West views on health and healing in the light of energy concepts. Reflexognosy will include discussions about all these disciplines and will work inter-professionally with these practitioners. Reflexognosy does have a base in energy medicine. For a practitioner, if he or she wants to make the shift in paradigm from the thought process of conventional tactile therapies and conventional medicine to reflexognosy and other wholistic disciplines will not be difficult.

Due to the fact that we stand at the threshold of the energy medicine frontier, it is not possible to give a definitive answer as to how reflexognosy works within energy medicine. It may be that the reflexognosist stimulates some intrinsic healing power which works with the life force of chi while working over acupuncture points, or innate intelligence of chiropractic, or with the vitalogy of a bygone era. But, for now, our attention needs to focus on the field of osteopathy. The theories of osteopathy will provide us with even more insights into how reflexognosy works on the physical level.

1 ___*Webster's New World Dictionary* (1988), pg. 643.

2 Evans, Michael & Lain Rodger. *Anthroposophical Medicine*, Thornsons, London, 1992, pgs. 59-66.

3 Williams, Tom. *Chinese Medicine*, Element Books, Great Britian, 1995, pg. 33.

4 Kaptchuk, Ted J. *The Web that has no Weaver*, Congdon & Weed, New York, 1983, pg. 142.

5 Gerber, Richard. *Vibrational Medicine*, Bear & Company, Santa Fe, New Mexico, 1988, pg. 125.

6 Ibid. pg. 124.

7 Ibid. pg. 125-126.

8 Grossman, Richard. *The Other Medicines*, Doubleday & Company, Inc. Garden City, New York, 1985, pg. 28.

9 Dold, Catherine. "Needles & Nerves", *Discover*, September 1998, pgs. 59-62.

10 Teegarden, Iona Marsha. *The Joy of Feeling, Bodymind Acupressure*, Japan Publications, New York, 1987, pg. 58.

11 Chopra, Deepak. *Perfect Health*, Harmony Books, New York, 1991, pg. 206

12 Hiss, John Martin. *Functional Foot Disorder*, The Oxford Press, Los Angeles, 1949, pgs. 135-136.

13 Ibid. pg. 135.

14 ___*The New Webster Encyclopedic Dictionary of the English Language*, pg. 289.

15 Tiller, William. Audio Tape *Energy Medicine 1* #6B, Edgar Foundation, 1983.

16 Gerber, pgs. 302-305.

17 Cornelius, Alfons. *Pressure Points, Their Origin and Significance,* Berlin, 1902. pg. 10.

18 Fitzgerald, William and Edwin Bowers. Zone Therapy, Health Research, Mokelumne Hill CA, 1917, pg. 15.

19 Gerber, pg. 346.

20 Riley, Joe Shelby. *Conquering Units: or the Mastery of Disease*, 1921, pg.8.

21 Riley, Joe Shelby and (Mrs.) L. Dow Balliett. *Numerology & Vibration,* Health Research, Mokelumne Hill, CA., 1959, pg. 4.

22 Ingham, Eunice. *Stories the Feet Have Told,* Ingham Publishing, St Petersburg, Florida, 1951, pg. 24.

23 Beal, Myron C.,"Osteopathic Basics", *Journal of the American Osteopathic Association*, Vol. 79. No. 7 March 1980, pg. 457.

POSSIBLE SHIFT IN PARADIGM

Conventional Tactile Therapies and Conventional Medicine	Reflexognosy™ and other Wholistic Disciplines
1. Based on Classical Physics' view: Cartesian/Newtonian	1. Based on Quantum Physics' view: Einstein/Bohr
2. Mechanistic view with cells, tissues, organs and glands as separate building blocks. In reflexology body is composed of points found on a foot chart.	2. Involves a process known as transaction—the simultaneous & mutually interdependent interaction between multiple components. No charts used, body cavities taught.
3. Follows medical model—Find and fix the problem or complaint.	3. Follows health model—Relaxation is a key, encourages body's own immune system.
4. Sees health as a lack of disease or symptoms in the physical body.	4. Sees illness & disease as congestion; and health as a continual balance between physical, mental, emotional and spiritual.
5. Strives to produce homeostasis of the body or body parts.	5. Belief in nature's inherent harmony. Balancing is a continual and dynamic process.
6. Works only physically through pressure to the nervous system by producing a reflex arc or action.	6. Wholistic disciplines working through the physical, the physiological, the mind, spiritually through the soul and subtle energy bodies.
7. The practitioner is a technician and his/her thoughts do not directly influence outcome.	7. The practitioner is part of the healing process, his/her thoughts influence outcome.

NOTE: Neither is right or wrong. Each paradigm is valid depending on the practitioner's perceptions, viewpoints, education and beliefs.

Chart 2

Chapter 6

Osteopathy & Reflexognosy

"The human body is a living machine that will run right so long as the anatomy or structural part of it is perfect."

—Andrew Still

Osteopathy was developed by Andrew Taylor Still in 1874 when he became dissatisfied with the medical practices of his day. Dr. Still served as a surgeon in the Union Army during the Civil War and later practiced as a 'bonesetter' [as early day chiropractors where called] in Kirksville, Missouri. It was in Kirksville that Still founded the American School of Osteopathy in 1892. Dr. Still developed the concept that the body's musculoskeletal system forms a structure that, when disordered, may effect changes in the function of other parts of the body. According to Dr. Still the body is a living machine that will run right so long as the anatomy or structural part of it is perfect. Yet osteopathy does not regard peculiarities of structure as strictly 'abnormal'. It assesses how the patient's structure has *adapted to the life it has led.* As the structure adapts this becomes the 'normal' for that body, with no ill effects. To Dr. Still the human body was an excellent example of adaptability.

Dr. Still also was a student of nature and pioneered the concept of preventive medicine by advising patients about eating right and keeping fit. Doctors of Osteopathy (D.O.) utilize a holistic approach and prefer treatments which stimulate the body's natural abilities to balance itself through manipulation of the spine, and palpation of reflexes and soft tissue. Edward Triance, D.O. (1986) writes, "Much vital energy is repressed by muscular tightness. This brings needless fatigue and tiredness, as muscle groups should be alternately tensed and relaxed."[1]

Eunice Ingham was a guest lecturer in the 1950s at the American School of Osteopathy. No doubt she was introduced to the concepts, if not through her own interests and research, then during her work at the clinic of the Osteopathic Hospital in St. Petersburg and her association with osteopath, Dr. Joe Shelby Riley in the mid-30s. Ingham refers to osteopathic and chiropractic concepts and research in *Stories The Feet*

Have Told (1951). Under a section titled 'Osteopathic Concept' Ingham writes, "A spinal lesion means an abnormal pull on muscle tissue. If we can release the excessive tension by contacting a specific reflex in the feet, we are helping to bring about a correction of that spinal lesion." [2]

In that statement Ingham combines two osteopathic concepts—lesions and reflexes.

Many other theories advanced in Osteopathy are of special interest to reflexognosists:

- "The freedom of circulation throughout the entire body is also only endured if the fascia is in an easy condition of tone. A healthy tone aids the muscles, ligaments and tendons which in turn aids the balance of the body. The condition of one is dependent upon the other and so the bones, muscles, tendons, ligaments and fascia act as a harmonizing team. [3]

- If there is fascial restriction this creates an energy restriction as well.

Both thoughts echo Ingham's oft repeated statement that, "Circulation is life and stagnation is death". [4]

Chapman's Reflexes

Another concept in Osteopathy is that of 'Chapman's Reflexes'. Chapman's reflexes are painful points discovered by Dr. Frank Chapman which are located all over the body that, when palpated, he felt could lead to the healing of disease.

Chapman's work was originally published in 1937 after his death. It was written by his co-researcher, Dr. Charles Owen. In the foreword to the 1963 reprinting—titled *An Endocrine Interpretation of Chapman's Reflexes by The Interpreter*, 2nd edition—Fred Mitchell, D.O. states, "Drs. Chapman and Owens were of the opinion that these reflexes were clinically useful in three principal ways:

1) for diagnosis;

2) for influencing the motion of fluids, mostly lymph; and

3) for influencing visceral [organ] function through the nervous system.

The relative constancy of the anatomic topography of Chapman's Reflexes makes it possible to establish the location of pathology without knowing its nature."[5] However, clearly defining what the word 'reflex' actually means is not established.

Mitchell records that Chapman felt by palpating the skin one could feel changes with the deep fascia. Changes, which often felt different when being palpated, were ganglioform contractions located at specific points and these points were consistently associated with different internal organs.

When Chapman entered the college in Kirksville in 1897 the prevailing thought was that there was no sickness without a bony lesion. A lesion, at that time, was defined as any abnormality in the structure of a tissue. The 'osteopathic lesion' was generally considered to be due to some form of strain resulting in a complete or partial fixation of a joint within its normal range of movement. However, thirty years of practice convinced Chapman that bony lesions accounted for only 20% of the health problems he encountered. Chapman would later expand on the definition by adding that structural change is accompanied by changes in the chemical structure and therefore the working conditions of the surrounding tissues.

In general, Chapman's Reflexes are found in *soft tissue* at various points along both sides of the sternum, the proximal head of humerus, distal and proximal clavicle, occipital ridge, cervicals, ribs, scapula, thoracics, lumbar, sacrum, coccyx, pelvis, pubis, fibula, and medial head of the tibia. Whether the location of these reflexes is either posterior, anterior, or both depends on the symptoms or complaints. When the condition involves an organ, then the location where the autonomic nerve ganglion branches off the spinal column to the organ, becomes one of the reflex points to be palpated.

Chapman, as part of the era of Vitalogy, found poor hygiene and diet responsible for the vast majority of problems. These lowered a person's vitality which in turn made him susceptible to viruses and infections. Poor hygiene and diet influenced bodily functions, particularly of the lymphatic system, causing blockages. Chapman wanted his colleagues to work with the lymphatic aspects of disease, regardless of the cause of the problem, clearing these blockages. He writes in the introduction of his work, "The ideas here presented respecting lymphatic reflexes have, to the best of my knowledge and belief, never been presented before."[6] Here Chapman seems to be referring to two different things: not only the lymphatic system but also to lymphatic reflexes.

What's a Reflex?

Reflexes, including Chapman's, are *not* objects. According to Mitchell, "Chapman's Reflexes is just a term given to these receptor organs because of the osteopath who discovered their diagnostic and therapeutic value in the location and treatment of disease."[7] Since Chapman's Reflexes were located all over the body the impression given was that a reflex is an object or point on the skin. At the same time palpation was thought to create a reflex action of some type.

Even contemporary osteopaths have difficulty in describing the concept of a reflex, it would appear that it is actually a physiological reaction and the osteopaths often interchange the terminology to include lesions. A lesion is an object that infers a restriction to soft tissue in the region of the spinal column, in particular the fascia. The term reflex is used as a kind of *slang* to describe the end result of a lengthy physiological process—a process, not an object. Lesion is the term used to describe the tactile sensation felt by the practitioner. However over the years the terms reflex and lesions have become synonymous. Ingham seems to have contributed her share to this misunderstanding by using the word reflex to describe a sensitive area while at the same time using it to also describe the physiological process produced by a reflex action.

To further confuse the issue, Chaitow notes in *Soft Tissue Manipulation* (1988) that 'reflexes' go by many names: Travell and associates refer to them as trigger points; Beal as viscerosomatic reflexes; Bennet as neurovascular points; Gutstein as myodysneuric points; Korr uses the terms facilitate segment and referred dysfunction; and in acupuncture they are *tsubo* points, yet all are discussing the same phenomena.

Regardless of the name, Chaitow classifies reflexes into one of three levels of responsive action.

- Level One. This is referred to as the sensory impulse known as a reflex arc. It should be noted that this impulse travels only as far as the spinal cord. In combination with a motor impulse an immediate muscle response is activated. This activation is termed a protective response.

- Level Two. This is the situation interpreted by the brain stem and is also protective in nature. Such activities as coughing and sneezing are examples of this kind of reflex.

- Level Three. Third level reflexes are learned or conditioned reflexes involving the cerebral cortex of the brain. Examples here include control of the bowel and bladder. An urge alerts the body to the need to urinate. This stimulus will prepare a person to void the bladder.

In all reflexes the essential structures involved are a receptor, an afferent neuron, a connecting neuron, an efferent neuron and an effector. Most reflex arcs involve hundreds of neurons, not a single physical point.

Dr. H.R. Small, who worked with Dr. Owens for four years, reported in 1937, on the relationship he discovered between Chapman's reflex to the spinal and sympathetic-nerves, pinpointing exactly where he

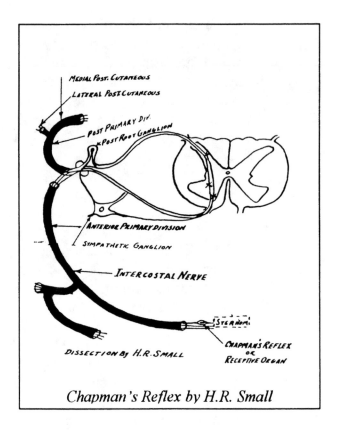

Chapman's Reflex by H.R. Small

locates the reflex. "In the intercostal space between the anterior and posterior layers of the anterior intercostal fascia is located some lymphoid tissue. It is within this tissue that a Chapman's reflex will be found. ...Stimulations of these receptor organs will cause the afferent and efferent vessels draining the tissues to increase or decrease, permitting the lymph flow to be increased or diminished, thus affecting the drainage of the entire lymph system of this area. Also through the sympathetic fibers of this tissue the lymph nodes of the vital organs (heart, kidneys, liver, spleen, pancreas, etc.) are affected. Chapman's Reflexes is just a term given to these receptor organs because of the osteopath who discovered their diagnostic and therapeutic value in the location and treatment of disease. Doubtless by consistently following the anatomy of this lymph system he was led to base his findings on purely anatomical research."[8]

This is very familiar to the thoughts put forth by Ingham over the years. It was this explanation that Ingham advanced in her work and first book about the meaning of sensitive areas found in the feet. The format of *Stories The Feet Have Told* parallels that of Chapman's work, *An Endocrine Interpretation of Chapman's Reflexes*. Explaining the results she obtained, Ingham said, "...try this simple method of producing a reflex action (by manipulation) through the nerve endings on the soles of the feet."[9] Here she is indicating a reflex action, then, like Chapman she produced charts that illustrated where points could be palpated to reach various organs and called them reflexes.

Techniques

The technique used to locate and work on an offending reflex was the pad of the middle or index finger. While gentle contact is maintained, a rotary motion is made. "The finger is not allowed to slip about, but is held firmly in contact with the locus"[10] [i.e., specific reflex point]. "Knowledge of the exact location of the reflex is paramount."[11] Chapman himself stressed that results would come more quickly and be less painful by gentle rather than strong pressure.

When discussing the 'dosage of treatment' Mitchell comments that the amount of treatment [i.e. application of pressure] would depend on the patient's physiological and chronological age; whether a symptom was

Reflex centers and notes for treating sinusitis according to Chapman.

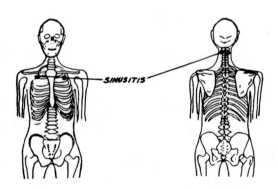

"A complete relaxation of both anterior and posterior contractions will completely relieve the above condition in a few days. This condition is almost invariably the result of faulty metabolism with its consequent accumulation of tissue waste. Except in cases where a marked endocrine disturbance exists, a few minutes treatment, skillfully applied to the reflexes, will frequently be accompanied with phenomenal results. It is not uncommon in such cases (even of several years standing that have resisted all previous treatment) to obtain permanent relief from two or three treatments, where reasonable care is exercised in their diet."[12]

acute or chronic, how much treatment the tissues can stand, and if there was any reaction to a previous treatment. "Over-treatment is possible in reflex work as in articular (joint) management."[13] The actual time a practitioner worked on a particular reflex could last from twenty seconds to two minutes or more. Mitchell stresses that over-treatment fatigued the reflex arc and nullified the good effect produced. However, he also cautioned that inefficient or insufficient work produced poor results. While admonishing the student to remember the inter-relationship of organ systems, he recommended working the system in the sequence it is found. For example, "work the distal colon before treating the proximal colon."[14]

Mitchell's quotes Lin Yutang, "A doctor who prescribes an identical treatment for an identical illness in two individuals and expects an identical development may be properly classified as a social menace," as a warning to the osteopathic practitioner not to treat all clients in the same way.

The 2nd edition of *Chapman's Reflexes* contains a foreword by 'The Interpreter'. It is not clear exactly who this mysterious interpreter is. However, the interpreter suggests when studying reflex work, the student:

1. Learn each reflex by *location rather than by sense of touch.* [emphasis by the interpreter]

2. Learn reflexes by groups (systems) one at a time; and

3. Learn to include the endocrine gland along with the nerve and

blood supply concerned in the disturbance.[15]

Learning each reflex by location and treating the location set a tradition in other disciplines—notably reflexology.

However, the authors would take exception to the advice given in point one, at least in connection with reflexognosy. We feel points of the body are unlikely to be precisely identifiable on the feet, but a general identification as to site is possible by thinking in terms of body cavities, areas of anatomical position or area rather than a specific point. It has been reported that one in ten thousand has his or her internal organs reversed. The solution, of course, is to work all surfaces of both feet thoroughly and let the body utilize the stimulation provided. Point two, learning reflexes in groups, or systems of the body, the authors concede does promote a more wholistic viewpoint rather than viewing parts of the body in isolation.

Endocrine Link

Two different systems coordinate the working of the body. The nervous system works by using electrical impulses, while the endocrine system uses chemicals called hormones.

Within the nervous system there are sensory neurons that carry nerve impulses from different parts of the body to the central nervous system. Some sensory neurons are directly triggered by stimuli while others are triggered indirectly, by special cells or neurons called receptors. Sensory neurons are plentiful in the soles of the feet.

Chapman's Reflexes demonstrated the connection of certain receptors to the endocrine system. If there is a lesion formed within the soft tissue of the spinal column then a stimulus by palpation will produce a reflex action that will in turn produce a physiological reaction to organs innervated from the autonomic nerve ganglia. The osteopathic inference is drawing from this influence on the spinal column. To this Chapman linked receptors and the role they play with the endocrine system. Communication does take place within the receptors and this could be why Chapman was the first to link the endocrinology of the body to the concept of reflexes. For the first time knowledge and treatment of the endocrine system comes under the scope of osteopathic practice.

Osteopathic Theory

Osteopathic theory proposes there is a direct relationship between disorders in joint motion and symptomatology. In many cases, there is a direct association with the return of function and the relief of symptoms.[16] In addition, in some way the autonomic nerve reflexes are involved in metabolic changes in soft tissues. It is not supposed that actual pressure on the body surface near the bony surface of the vertebrae is the underlying cause of a disease as in chiropractic. Osteopathy is not usually used in the treatment of infectious diseases although it may be used in conjunction with other treatment because of its effect on the sympathetic nervous system, the circulation, and hormone secretion.

Similarly, osteopathy cannot directly relieve organic diseases in which the structure of the organs is affected, however, it may be of benefit when it improves the tone of muscles, relieves tension, and restores relaxation as "...any constriction or congestions will interfere with the vital processes and normal functions of the body tissues. ...The zone of the spine from which the nerves emerge which are concerned with any particular organ or area of the body must be specially considered in osteopathic treatment."[17] [Note the usage of the term zone in the preceding statement.]

Osteopathy's Connection to the Feet

An interesting point to consider in Chapman's work is that nowhere are the feet or hands involved as sites to be worked. However, we do know that sensory neurons are plentiful in the soles of the feet. From the previous remarks it appears that Chapman's Reflexes are objects, and their description would coincide with the reflexologists' description of points they find and work in the feet. Dr. Joe Shelby Riley, may have reached this same conclusion and adapted Chapman's concept, which he knew about through his own osteopathic training, to the feet and hands while coupling reflexes with Fitzgerald's work with zones. Riley's charts are the oldest which map the various 'reflex' points on the feet. Riley's work was further refined and popularized by Ingham who worked as his assistant for several months during two successive winters in Florida and, as previously mentioned, also worked in the clinic of an Osteopathic Hospital.

With Chapman's concepts in

mind, the feet may support much the same principles. First, sensitivity in the soft tissue of the foot, [e.g. pain upon palpatory pressure] may affect the body as the fascia forms lesions and adversely affects biomechanical movement. Additionally, the proper alignment of the joint produces relief of tension to the segmental dysfunction of the dermatomes resulting in the relaxation of tension—muscular and nervous—throughout the body and the reduction of pain as normalization of receptor activity moves toward normal muscle tone. The relaxation process will reverberate up the spinal column and through the autonomic nerve ganglia to the organs and other parts of the body due to the close ties between the central nervous system and the autonomic nervous system. The result of palpation to the receptors on the feet coupled with joint activation produce the range of reactions seen in reflexognosy.

For this reason we cannot isolate our thinking to the concept that pressing one reflex point on the foot will directly influence only the area of the body that the reflex point is thought to represent. Stimulus travels at enormous speeds and involves very diverse areas of the body. Removal of articular lesions coupled with the hormonal activation triggering an endocrine response, stimulation to the circulatory and lymphatic systems, and all nervous systems makes reflexognosy a very powerful and wholistic therapy.

Ingham (1951) puts it more simply in *Stories the Feet Have Told* by saying, "If any degree of tenderness is found in those reflexes in that part of the foot relative to the spine,

then by applying this form of compression massage to that area you will relax the muscle tension surrounding that vertebra."[18] In fact, the actual processes the practitioner has affected includes:

- structure alignment which produces
- reduced tension on the fascia that may result in
- improved circulation and
- pain reduction
- improving overall health.

Dr. Fred Mitchell also says that "bizarre combinations of reflexes may be impossible to explain with our present knowledge. Treat what you find...not what you are looking for!"[19]

Palpatory Terminology

Before leaving osteopathy and its connection to reflexognosy let us look briefly at the terminology used by osteopaths when examining the texture of tissue under their fingers and the subject of pressure. Typically palpation involves both the use of light-touch and deep-touch to discover changes taking place in the skin and subcutaneous tissue. Light touch can either be passive, where the fingers rest lightly on the skin, or active whereby the fingers move from site to site. Beal (1980) states "In deep-touch, the fingers compress the skin surface, palpating through skin and subcutaneous tissues to the superficial muscle. Further compression leads to palpation of deeper muscles, fascia, and bone. Deep palpation utilizes forces of compression and shear. Compression is a force applied perpendicularly to the skin surface. Shear is a force applied parallel to the skin surface. In some instances, deep palpation combines both compression and shear in the exploration of deep tissue texture."[20] Note the use of the term compression—the same word which at one time Eunice Ingham used to describe her work as 'the reflex method of compression massage' before finally settling on the term reflexology. From this it is clear, the techniques, and nomenclature employed by reflexologists and reflexognosists are closely aligned with osteopathic principles and 'reflexes' not those of massage as some would claim.

To reflexognosy Osteopathy contributes:

- The importance of structural integrity

- The terms and theories of reflexes, lesions and compression

- The importance of the autonomic nerve ganglion innervating the organs and endocrine system

- Tactile skills and soft tissue manipulation of 'reflexes'

- A wholistic approach to illness utilizing diet, hygiene and touch.

Osteopathic theory and techniques provide one piece of the puzzle as to why dynamic changes occur in reference to working on the legs and feet. Both Chiropractic and Osteopathy look to problems or malalignments in the spinal area as the cause for illness in the rest of the body. Neither profession concentrates heavily on the feet. However, structural deviation from normalcy in the feet can be the foundation of spinal lesions and subluxations which in turn have an affect on the entire body. With this concept in mind, the importance of the role of feet in health will be our next focus.

---

[1] Triance, Edward. *Osteopathy*, Thorsons Publishing Group, Wellingborough, England, 1986 pg 65-66.

[2] Ingham, Eunice. *Stories the Feet Have Told*, Ingham Publishing, St. Petersburg, Florida, 1951, pg. 30.

[3] Triance, pgs 60-61.

[4] Ingham, Eunice. *Stories the Feet Can Tell*, Ingham Publishing, St. Petersburg Florida, 1938, pg. 98, 109.

[5] The Interpreter. *An Endocrine Interpretation of Chapman's Reflexes*, 6th printing, American Academy of Osteopathy, Newark Ohio, 1992, pg. iii.

[6] Ibid. pg. v.

[7] Ibid. pg. 2.

[8] Ibid. pg. 2.

[9] Ingham, *Stories the Feet Can Tell*, pg. Introduction.

[10] The Interpreter, pg. iii.

[11] Ibid. pg. iii

[12] Ibid. pg. 38.

[13]c Ibid. pg. iii.

[14] Ibid. pg. iv.

[15] Ibid. pg. 3.

[16] ____ *Virtue's Household Physician* pg. 889-892.

[17] Beal, Myron, C. "Osteopathic Basics", *Journal of the American Osteopathic Association* Vol. 79. No 7 March 1980, pg. 458.

[18] Ingham, pg. 30-31

[19] The Interpreter, pg. iv.

[20] Beal, Myron, C. pg. 457.

Chapter 7

The Role of Feet in Health

When things aren't going so neat
Remember the legs and the feet

—**William Schultz**

D r. Hiss (1938) leads us in this debate and eludes to the wholistic value of the feet. "About 90% of the shoes made today disturb the delicate balance of the feet, to the extent that they cannot withstand the jars and mis-steps, incident to walking on the hard sidewalks of our modern civilization. Foot function is upset. All this results in either tension, or locking of the joints, strain in the muscles, limitation of foot motion, or a combination of all of these. The direct consequence is discomfort—aches and pains in the feet, legs, knees, thighs and back"[1] This quote indicates the importance of the feet in health and is still true today, half a century after it was written.

As the foundation of a house settles, cracks frequently appear in the walls and ceilings as a result of stress that is transmitted to these structures from the shifting or settling of the foundation below. In a similar way, man's feet comprise his foundation.

When they are well, they serve; when sick, they cause pain. Structural fault in the feet transmit stress to the joints and muscles of the entire body, causing aches and pains in the feet and elsewhere. Yet the important aspects the feet play in the body and in overall health are often overlooked.

This was not always the case however. Although not an the area of actual treatment, in the late 1920s and through the 1930s within osteopathy, there was an emphasis on the relationship between the feet, shoes, and overall health. The concept was so popular that shoe companies published their own booklets which covered foot manipulation, shoe fitting, and foot exercises.

Dr. B.C. Maxwell (1936) felt that the condition of the feet affected the personality and the remainder of the body because his finding indicated, "...so intimately are the feet connected, back and forth, with the central nervous system".[2]

The action of the knee, hip

and other parts of the body are dependent on the foot. Goldthwait et al, in *Body Mechanics in Health and Disease* state: "The foot plays an extremely important part in the mechanics of the whole body. In a discussion of hygiene or of the treatment of disabilities it should not be considered separately from the rest of the body."[3] According to the above authors, who are all medical doctors, one of the most common causes of foot deformity is a result of anatomic changes. These changes are seen in the bones, muscles, and ligaments as an outgrowth or end result of weakness where permanent shortening or weakening of muscles or ligaments has come from long persistence in a faulty position or with a disease which may lead to limitation of motion and deformity such as arthritis.

Another disturbance, more commonly seen in individuals past midlife, is impairment of function from circulatory disturbances. Write Goldthwait et al, "Here, while the exciting cause may be any one of a large number of conditions which can disturb function of the heart, arteries, or veins, bad body mechanics plays a very important part in its development. ...In impairment of function from circulatory disturbance, complete recovery can be expected in milder cases with the development of good body mechanics as the only form of treatment. ...In the care of deformity, where structural change has occurred in the foot, attempts must be made to secure as nearly normal a position for function as possible."[4]

According to Clybourne (1931), foot ailments can play a large part in breaking down of the body with resulting symptomatology.[5]

Anatomically the feet are important in venous and lymphatic return from the leg, as the pumping action in the gastroc-soleus muscles requires active plantar flexion and dorsiflexion of the ankle, plus flexion and extension of the knee, and leg elevation. The techniques selected by a reflexognosist will include assessment of these actions and offer a treatment plan.

Podiatrist Howard J. Danaberg, DPM (1994) believes the foot is the basis of many pain related problems in other parts of the body. "If the foot is not operating properly, the gait will be affected. Since most of us take thousands of steps every day, an out-of-wack gait can cause adaptations and adjustments in the body that can cause pain in the knees, hip, back, even the head and jaw."[6] R. Daryl Phillips DPM, (1994) Professor of Podiatric Medicine at the University of Osteopathic Medicine and Health Sciences College of Podiatric Medicine and Surgery, Des Moines Iowa, comments in the same article, "There are many anecdotal stories about pain reduction or elimination in distant parts of the body due to correction of foot or gait problems...."[7] Reflexognosy takes a further step in this concept and includes organ function and the entire anatomy of the foot (see Chapter 8) itself by questioning the stress placed on the body as the foot deviates from normalcy. Structural deviation from normalcy within the foot will affect the foot and gait directly and the rest of the body indirectly.

The Work of Dr. Simon Wikler

A human walking and standing is totally dependent on their feet.

For this reason Dr. Simon Wikler (1911-1991), an American podiatrist often said, "The foot is a mechanical marvel. It acts as a short flexible rod that must support, propel, and provide hundreds of postural combinations for the huge body above it. To distort and weaken the foot causes mechanical stressful havoc to the entire body." [8] Wikler felt the foot is one of the most complex organs in the human body. According to him the foot is meant to move in more than 150 different ways so it can easily pronate, supinate and aid the body in assuming many postural positions. Wikler believed if the feet are seriously aberrated it leads to constant and unrelenting stresses and strains throughout the body. In turn, constant stress is an acknowledged predisposition to unknown causes of some cancers, degenerative and chronic diseases.

"The distortions and weaknesses of the feet in shape, movement, strength and muscle density shows us the predisposition to certain deadly diseases," [9] Wikler commented during a lecture before reflexologists in 1990 in Toronto. Studies he conducted at the University of Pretoria, South Africa, Coronary Rehabilitation Clinic and Ohio State University Comprehensive Cancer Center, both in 1987, showed a statistical relationship between shoe distorted feet and coronary disease, as well as cancer of the breast in women.

"I am not claiming every American woman with poor feet is going to get cancer of the breast. However, one out of ten does get it. The Comprehensive Cancer Center of the Ohio State University with whom I did a study with 200 subjects found, to their surprise, that women with breast cancer have poorer feet than women without breast cancer," [10] Wikler declared.

Wikler developed for his research studies a nine-point foot evaluation protocol. He measured such things as outer toe strength, toe spreading, toe deformity, hip rotation, the presence of a bunion, pronation, calf contraction, muscle depth on the bottom of the foot, and shoulder posture. Each was important for a different biomechanical reason. All the muscles of the foot have to do with bending the toes and the ability to spread the toes enables a person to keep the entire body in easy balance. Any toe deformity and inefficiencies throws the mechanics of the entire body off and puts the body under stress. Wikler predicted that statistics will eventually reveal that what we do to our toes is as dangerous to our health as bacteria is. Reflexognosists have refined Wikler's nine-point evaluation and find it remarkable as an aid to developing a treatment plan.

Wikler justified his position by saying, "Walking is an effortless exercise if the calf muscles are supple. Unless one can take a long stride while the other heel is still on the ground that stride will be stressful. A bunion causes the leverage action of the foot to diminish and this leads to fatigue when standing or walking. When a step is taken the hip plays a very important part. The heavy musculature of the buttocks and thighs when properly moved, have a bearing on the big heavy, thick pelvic arteries, the femoral and common iliac, which supply the limbs with large amounts of blood. When the thigh and hip do not function correctly the biomechanical function is affected throwing off the gait and impeding peripheral vascular circulation. For women, shoulder posture is especially important because of the incidence of breast cancer. When women wear high heels they throw their posture off and round their shoulders. This causes the breast, instead of hanging from the strong tissues, as slings, from the collar and breast bones, to hang more from the weak tissue of the armpits. This results in constant injury to the upper outside of the breast which happens to be the common site of initial cancers of the breast."[11]

Wikler wrote his first article on foot trouble as the cause of cancer of the breast in 1950. The article was published as "Foot Defects as Possible Etiological Factors in Cancer", in the *Journal of the National Association of Chiropodists*, August 1950. The following year he published "Hypothetical Relationship of Foot Imbalance to Rheumatic Fever" in the same journal. Over the years he also visited many countries and studied thousands of feet, finding that people who had a resistance to heart disease and breast cancer habitually either went bare footed or wore non-deforming shoes. Three subsequent books were written by Dr. Wikler on this theory. He also designed a special shoe for children so their feet would not needlessly be distorted. Ten million pairs of non-deforming shoes for children known as the Wikler Shoe, manufactured by the Buster Brown Shoe Company, were sold around the world. In spite of his commercial success, the academic world did not pursue his theories or fund any studies.

Finally, in 1987, nearly forty years after his initial article was published, some interest was shown

which allowed Dr. Wikler to do two relatively small scale, blind studies. The first was at the South African University of Pretoria in the Kalfong Hospital. Here, in a few days, Dr. Wikler saw approximately two hundred people half of whom had coronary disease and half of whom did not. A cardiologist, Dr. M. W. Loock was assigned to sit next to him to make sure Wikler said nothing to the subjects as he took five minutes to evaluate each person's feet. From these evaluations he picked the ones with poorer feet as the ones who had heart trouble. To the surprise of Dr. Loock, Wikler was right! Writes Wikler of the experience, "This came as no surprise to me. I had observed this in forty years of practice."[12]

That same year Drs. John Minton and David Yahn of the Ohio State University Comprehensive Cancer Center invited Wikler to do a foot evaluation of approximately two hundred women who were patients of Dr. Minton's. Some had cancer of the breast and others did not. Dr. Yahn sat alongside Wikler to make sure he asked no questions which would give him any clues as to the patients' condition. The results were the same. Dr. Yahn, wanting to enlarge the study, sent letters to breast surgeons and x-ray clinics where large groups of women were assembled who had breast cancer. To Wikler's disappointment permission was never granted that would have allowed him to do a simple, non-invasive visual assessment study. The reason given was that it would upset the women.

Dr. Wikler was asked to put his theory to the test through two research studies and proved them to be correct. He looked at women's forefeet and was able to identify the ones that had mammary disturbances, or chest problems.

From a podiatrist's perspective he observed the frontal plane disturbance of the foot and the more

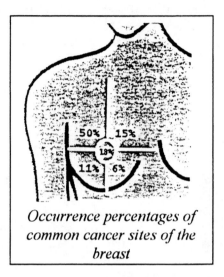

Occurrence percentages of common cancer sites of the breast

disturbed it was through bunions, hammer toes, or excessive supination or pronation, the more the front of the body would be adversely affected. In other words, for Dr. Wikler, if anything affects the frontal plane, the body is thrown forward restricting circulation to the axillary section of the body. The transference of toxins coming through the axillary lymph would not take place, congesting the anterior or frontal plane. His studies have indicated the strong possibility that the concept of somatic replication of the forefoot may have scientific validity. He felt, from a podiatrist's point of view, that the feet and locomotion influenced body function.

Reflexognosists owe Dr. Wikler a tremendous debt of gratitude. Beyond a doubt his studies prove the relationship that exists between the forefoot and the body. They scientifically validate the concept of somatic replication of the

body's cranial and thoracic cavities on the forefoot. He also introduces the possible marriage of reflexognosy, podiatry, and biomechanics.

Human beings are not machines. The body performs machine like functions but that does not mean it is a machine. Our feet do more than just propel us and hold the body upright. Our feet are a vital part of our body and it appears they are the foundation of our health also. When a person does not locomote in a balanced way, the body becomes rigid, stressing the entire anatomical structure and producing congestion. As demonstrated by Wikler, if the feet are biomechanically unsound the whole body is 'thrown off balance'. This stress factor may manifest as a sore back, sore ankles, knees, hips, neck or jaw. In addition to structural importance, the feet also house a rich nerve, arterial, and venous supply which influences other parts of the body. Linked with this major supply of blood are the dermatomes. Moreover energy channels and meridians in the feet link up with all parts of the body. Disturbances in energy fields also cause illness.

As wholistic practitioners the reflexognosist has a mind-body focus, or a whole person-whole foot focus. Applying pressure to the feet creates a reaction to all parts of the body and restores energy flow helping the body to revitalize. Toes have a distinct function, biomechanically and with energy. We get the results we do through the:

- meridians

- chakras

- subtle energy

- anatomy

- biomechanics

- nerve receptors

- fascia, and

- touch.

Not because we are pushing points on the feet.

Foot health has a direct link to the health of the body. We must search for cause and effect. Structural deviations will do this. Through structural analysis and skillful hands-on application of techniques we affect every part of the body. The foot is the foundation to good health and as the deviations from normalcy occur this will stress the body. The greater the deviations the more stress will be placed on the body resulting in the possibility of ill health. Validation for this hypothesis has been proven by a trial with podiatry and reflexognosy. A research study conducted by the Global Reflexognosy Research Institute of Professionals and reported at the 1993 International Council of Reflexologists Conference held in Melbourne, Australia confirmed that deviations from normalcy in the feet had a bearing on organ and skeletal function. The greater the deviation from normalcy the greater presentation of dysfunction.[13]

There is a rich, vibrant profession waiting to be created for professional foot assessors, as reflexognosists. Professionals who know the foot, understand its function, and the foot's importance in health. As a foundation, anatomy must be studied and learned well. Anatomy deals with cold hard facts.

There is no speculation, it is an exact science. With restriction of movement—rigidity develops, structure changes, and conditions occur. The role of the feet in health is critical as our health is affected with every step we take. In the next chapter we will take a closer look at the foot as an organ of the body.

---

[1] Hiss, John Martin. *"Treatment and care of Feet"*, lecture at Columbia University 1938, pg. 1.

[2] Maxwell, B.C. *Two Feet of Foot Comfort Through Self-Exercising*, Cleveland, Ohio, 1936, pg. 6.

[3] Goldthwait, Brown, Saim, and Kuhns *Body Mechanics in Health and Disease*, 3rd Edition, J.B. Lippincott, Co., Philadelphia pg. 262.

[4] Ibid. pg. 265-267.

[5] Clybourne, Harold E. Columbus Ohio, *Journal AOA*, February 1931, pg. 262.

[6] Danaberg, Howard J. "The Foot's The Thing" *Prevention*, December 1994, pg. 116.

[7] Ibid. pg. 118.

[8] Wikler, Simon and Christine Issel. Unpublished manuscript, "A Cause and Prevention of Breast Cancer and Heart Disease is at Hand", 1990, pg. 15.

[9] Wikler, *A Guide to Foot Assessment for Reflexologists*, Sacramento CA, 1990, pg. 2.

[10] Ibid. pg. 3.

[11] Wikler & Issel, pg. 10.

[12] Wikler & Issel, pg. 3

[13] Rogers, Sandra. "Reflexology on Trial", *LifeWise: The Australian Journal of Natural Therapies and Allied Health Care*, Vermont, Victoria, Vol. 1 No. 4, December 1993, pg.17

Chapter 8

The Foot as a Foot

"Feet are like faces—No two of them alike."
—John Martin Hiss

Anatomy does not change, but our understanding of anatomy and its clinical significance does change as does anatomical terminology and nomenclature. To the reflexognosist the foot has a double function. There is the foot involving somatic replication, which explains the results, and the foot as a foot, an *organ* of the body. Though not commonly thought of as an organ, the foot is a part of the body composed of specialized tissues and is adapted to the performance of specific functions. Seen in this light the foot is a most complicated organ. It is designed to move in over 200 directions. The 26 bones of the foot—1/4 of all the bones in the body—are held together by 107 ligaments and 19 muscles. It is also a sensory organ. Messages fly back and forth from the brain as to the position of the body in space, balance, and movement.

From the Reflexognosy perspective, the healthy foot is a re-flection of health. If the foot is pliable and firm the body attached to it is most likely in a similar healthy condition. In addition, the reflexognosist is aware that pain in the foot means a problem in the delicate anatomy of the foot.

As an organ the foot is designed to perform the following functions:

- Support the body

- Balance the body in space and compensate for changing positions in response to terrain

- Move the body through space

- Distribute the body's loading through the foot with each step

- Transform chemical energy into mechanical/kinetic energy

- Provide sensory reception to our body in terms of space, walking surface, and sensations of pressure, pain, and temperature

- Help sustain the body's vitality through it's contribution to the lymph and circulatory systems

- Act as a response mechanism through the Central Nervous System

The foot is a mobile, weight bearing structure. The large tarsal bones and short phalanges relate to this function. The bony structure, is reinforced and maintained by ligaments and tendons which articulate at the tarsal and phalangeal joints and influence the muscles. They assist the foot to dorsiflex and plantarflex, and form arches—the transverse, lateral and medial [longitudinal]. Arches are important in absorbing shock loads and balancing the body. The longitudinal arch transmits the force of body weight to the ground when standing and to the great toe in locomotion, creating a giant lever that provides spring to the gait. It is therefore very important to a reflexognosist, to assist in maintaining structural alignment in the feet. This can be achieved by foot activation techniques. When the bones of the feet are seated correctly, the client is able to achieve good energy stimulation, blood flow, and the nerves are able to function more efficiently. The feet are constructed of skin, muscles, tendons, ligaments, nerves, bones, blood vessels, and lymphatic nodes. Like any other part of the body, exercise can provide stimulation, strengthening and flexibility.

Scope of Practice for the Reflexognosist: Leg & Foot

Reflexognosists move be-yond the ankle knowing that the movement of the foot and toes is controlled by the muscles in the leg. When there is tenderness or spasms within the muscles of the leg it can cause the foot to behave in an abnormal way affecting the whole body. Gently stimulating the legs can increase circulation and release pressure in the foot as reflexognosy provides an effective dual application.

On uneven surfaces, muscles in the anterior [front] of the leg assist the body to stand in balance, despite the surfaces. At other times tight leg muscles can create a poor heel strike and foot curve, causing improper weight distribution to the medial or lateral side of the foot. Tight muscles in the posterior compartment [calf] can cause inefficient shock absorption adding strain or pain to the intrinsic anatomy of the foot. This may result in a vibratory jolt to the knees, hips, lower back moving up to the shoulders, neck and head. When the ankles lose strength and flexibility, the impact of locomotion sends vibrations to the metatarsals and the toes. In response, the toes can either be dorsiflexed or plantarflexed, and the energy for propulsion is greatly reduced.

A reflexognosist will focus on obtaining a flexible action in the feet. This will change the appearance of the foot. Photographic and imprint records of the feet are important and should be part of a client's record so as to document these changes. Usually the look of the foot will change within six sessions, particularly if there has been prescribed a combination of foot and leg exercises.

Reflexognosy provides both stimulation and sensory input through touch and movement of the foot. The ability of the foot to move to its full range of movement is of vital importance. Relaxation techniques are of equal importance. They have their own therapeutic function and play a key role in the healing process and must precede the more advanced techniques. Relaxation techniques also provide valuable information to the practitioner about the needs to be met in a treatment plan.

Anatomy of the Foot

A study of foot anatomy reveals:

- Bones—26 + 2 sesamoids, approximately one fourth of all bones in the body

- Musles/tendons/ligaments—17 intrinsic muscles within the foot, 107 ligaments and 12 tendons

- Nerves

- Fascia

- Connective tissue

- Blood supply

While the tendons connect bone to muscle, the ligaments serve three functions:

1. to hold bones in place

2. aid in movement and

3. connect bones to each other

When a ligament is not doing its job the muscles takes over, the muscle or tendon thickens and/or hardens, and is usually sensitive to the touch. Upon tactile examination, the reflexognosist determines if the area of sensitivity is radiating from the muscle, the bone, or some other tissue.

Sections of the Foot

The foot's importance cannot be stressed enough because practically all activity in life begins with foot function. In order to be able to understand the components which make up the biomechanical movement of the feet it is necessary to review the sections of the feet.

The first section is the tarsus. This is also known as the rear foot, or hindfoot, and includes the talus and the calcaneus.

Section two is referred to as the lesser tarsus or more commonly known as the mid-foot. The bones found in this section are the cuboid, navicular and cuneiforms.

Section three is comprised of the metatarsals (1-5) with the medial metatarsal being number one. It also includes the sesamoids.

Between sections two and three is the tuberosity of the 5th metatarsal.

Section four is the phalanges, numbered one to five, from the medial to the lateral. They are composed of two or three bones with the ones closest [proximal] to the metatarsals being called the proximal phalanges. Toes 2-5 have mid or intermedial phalanges. The end bones are called distal phalanges. It is not unusual for those phalanges to be fused. Sometimes one will find the phalanges in different positions as joints move out of place. Some in a state of abduction while others will be adducting.

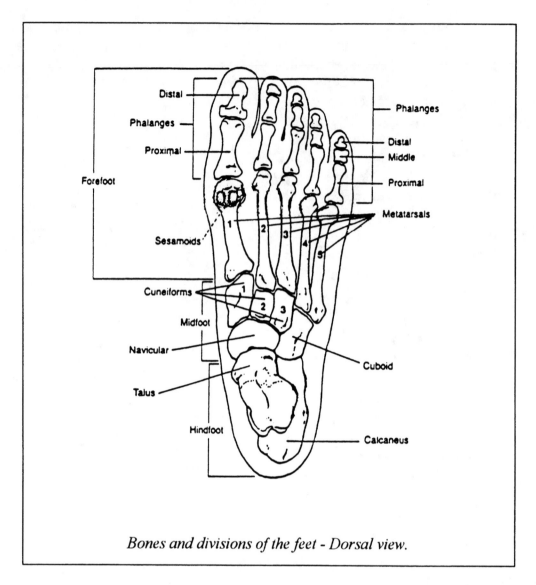

Bones and divisions of the feet - Dorsal view.

Normally, the phalanges fit squarely on the distal end of the metatarsals, forming the metatarsophalangeal joints.

All of these sections must move in unison during locomotion for correct foot curve. If they do not then the energy of the body is thrown completely out of 'balance'. The actual balance of the skeletal framework is somewhat impaired and then physiological problems may develop. In other words, structural normalcy in the foot provides the framework for balance and stress reduction to the me-

chanical movements of the body. If biomechanical disorders are not rectified, structural deviations will prevent Reflexognosy from being as successful as it could be.

The Phalanges

Phalanges refer to the bones of the toes, whereas digit refers to the whole toe. The digits play an important role to the foot and indirectly to the whole body. They are vital in providing balance and flow when standing and walking. If one works on the Eastern philosophy that there are energy meridians

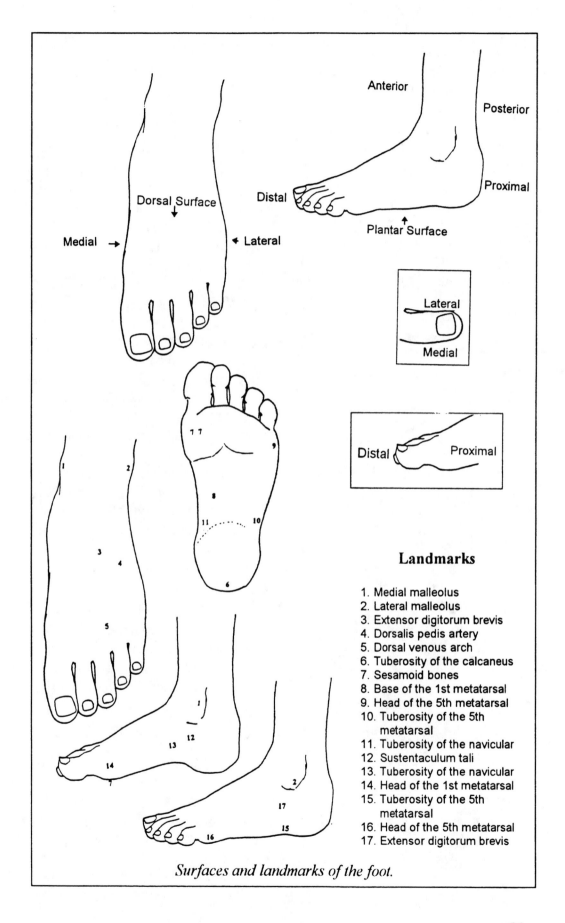

Surfaces and landmarks of the foot.

Landmarks

1. Medial malleolus
2. Lateral malleolus
3. Extensor digitorum brevis
4. Dorsalis pedis artery
5. Dorsal venous arch
6. Tuberosity of the calcaneus
7. Sesamoid bones
8. Base of the 1st metatarsal
9. Head of the 5th metatarsal
10. Tuberosity of the 5th metatarsal
11. Tuberosity of the navicular
12. Sustentaculum tali
13. Tuberosity of the navicular
14. Head of the 1st metatarsal
15. Tuberosity of the 5th metatarsal
16. Head of the 5th metatarsal
17. Extensor digitorum brevis

running the length of the body including the feet and toes, then the effect on a person not having a proper gait may affect the flow of vital energy. Toes that are not structurally sound cannot perform their important tasks efficiently.

To a reflexognosist, toes are an integral part of a session. It is important to work over the dorsal and plantar aspects of the phalanges as well as working between the toes, moving toward the metatarsophalangeal joints. Working around the distal aspect of each toe is also of benefit to the outcome of the overall session due to the at-

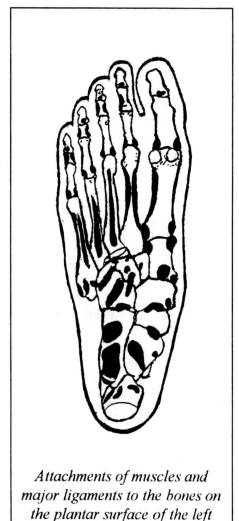

Attachments of muscles and major ligaments to the bones on the plantar surface of the left foot.

tachment of tendons to them and the meridians housed on the dorsal aspect.

Landmarks of the Feet

The landmarks of the feet are also important to the reflexognosist. They often do more than relate to somatic replication guidelines. For instance the tuberosity of the 5th metatarsal is one of the features that is a support mechanism for correct foot curve. It is also important for balance. Landmarks are points of visual recognition for the anatomy and tactile awareness and determine what type of work or techniques are in order. As an example, if the 1st metatarsal and the first cuneiform are out of place the client will have a bump on the dorsum of the foot and joint activation will be called for. In addition, the language of landmarks helps us describe to other professionals, the area we are finding sensitive through the use of common terminology.

Muscles

The muscles of the legs and feet are very important to reflexognosists for many reasons. First, as mentioned previously, most of the muscles in the feet have their origin in the legs, therefore if one wishes to relax the feet the place to start is in the legs. Second, many of the areas that are found to be sensitive and often regarded as reflex points, are the insertion points of muscles and ligaments. Furthermore, these painful areas can also be points of attachments of the ligaments and tendons. Relieving the stress on the origin and insertion points of the muscles will often release sensitivity when it is found. The third thing to consider is the biomechanical function of the muscles. In the event that something is interfering with proper gait, the muscles will suffer stress and be tender to the touch.

Arches

The longitudinal arch is one that runs along the medial aspect of the foot. We have an inner longitudinal arch and an outer longitudinal arch. Both of those arches provide support to the transverse section of the foot. We also have a transverse arch. In addition to support, arches contribute shock absorption. Shock absorption, in turn, promotes balance.

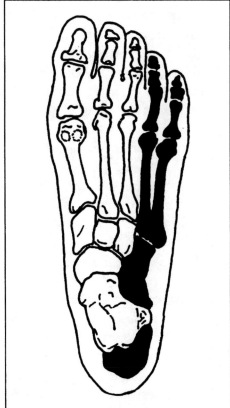

The medial side of the foot is for shock absorption, while the lateral side is designed for balance.

The Foot As A Sensory Organ

Through the traditional five senses—sight, hearing, touch, taste and smell—the body is aware of what is going on in the world around it. The body is equipped with sense organs, sensitive to the various kinds of energy in the environment. Without these organs, which collect this energy and translate it into nerve impulses which are then transmitted to the brain where they are interpreted, all links with the environment would be lost. The eyes receive and convert energy in the form of light. The ears receive and convert energy in the form of sound. The skin is sensitive to energy arriving at the body as temperature, pressure and touch. Chemical changes at the tongue and nose induce electrical changes which are finally translated as taste and smell. Sense organs only use a tiny proportion of the information which floods into them.

The sense organs are confined to a small part of the body. Excluding the skin, whose surface has an enormous number of sensory receptors receiving stimuli of heat, cold, touch and pain, the largest sensory organ is the foot which is not conventionally thought of as a sense organ. The foot has many perceptional abilities in common with other sense organs. Like the ears it is concerned with balance; like the eyes, it judges distance. Of course it perceives all the sensations of touch, and indirectly, through absorption of aromatic and therapeutic substances in the forms of herbal infusions and essential oils, it has something in common with the senses of smell and taste.

The sensory input from the foot provides the body with the ability to receive information about its position in space and in movement. This is called proprioception. Proprioceptors [the actual nerve cells] occur chiefly in muscles, tendons and the inner ear, which initially perceives the position to the rest of the body so that posture is maintained by unconscious reflex movements as the body adjusts to the stimulation. The foot also perceives the texture of the surface it is in contact with. This includes assessing factors such as contour evenness, temperature, and safety. Is the area slippery or steep? Locomotion variations occur by adjustments in stride, pressure, stretch and movement.

Direct pressure to the soles of the feet is interpreted by the brain as pressure and the brain loosens the muscles in response. When the pressure has stopped, the muscles can return to a more relaxed state. In this way the stimulation provided by reflexognosy aids in reprogramming a greater range of motion and a more natural step. At the same time, in response to the pressure, the oxygen and nutrients needed by the muscle groups throughout the body are sent, even though these muscles are not actively working. Reflexognosy acts as a means of varying sensory experience and encouraging flexibility, not only to the foot but also to the internal environment via improved peripheral vascular return and circulatory stimulation.

Besides receiving and transmitting stimuli to the brain, the sense organs provide built-in protection against excessive energy input through the sensation of pain. The sense of touch serves to provide a warning of danger for the body. Anything which causes a sensation of pain is also likely to cause damage to the body's tissues and immediate action is called for to avoid injury. Although the signals in nerve fibers move rapidly, painful stimuli tend to bring about a reflex response. With reflexognosy, when sensitivity is discovered as a reflex response, a message from the toe or foot reaches the spinal cord and from here messages are passed directly to a muscle group, which brings about a withdrawal of the foot, in fact, before the brain becomes aware of the pain.

The region of the brain where sensations of temperature, pain, and touch are perceived is the sensory cortex of the parietal lobe. There is a crossover in the pathways of sensation from the body before the brain is reached. The sensory nerves cross either in the spinal cord or in the brain stem so that sensations from the left side of the body reach the sensory cortex of the right cerebral hemisphere and those from the right side of the body are registered in the left cortex.

Each region of the body sends signals that reach a fairly well-defined area of the sensory cortex and as a result of experiments it has been possible to map out the cortex to show the area of the body represented. (See sensory homunculus illustration in Chapter 2.) The toes are nearest the fissure between the left and right hemispheres. Passing to the side and downward are the terminations of the pathways from the leg, trunk, arm, hand, face, tongue throat and the internal organs. The parts of the body represented with the greatest sensitivity are represented by the largest areas of sensory cortex, so the fingers, thumbs, and lips are each represented by almost as large an area as the rest of the body put together. The strip of sensory cortex in one hemisphere is duplicated in the other hemisphere.

The condition of the foot is also a barometer of the body. By taking the pulse at the dorsal pedis artery an insight about the constitution of the body can be drawn. The existence of diabetes, Raynauds Syndrome, intermittent claudication and nutritional deficiencies can be determined through the color and temperature of the feet. Presence of wounds that will not heal and the existence of certain nail conditions will provide information that will be of clinical assistance.

The foot is one of the most important sensory stimulators and receptors found in the body. The foot is a sensory organ and since no part of the body is in isolation from any other, it works with the functioning of the rest of the body. Pressure on the lateral edge of the foot is perceived by the body in a certain way and a reaction occurs to maintain the position of the body. The foot specializes in the information which results in locomotion, with each step it communicates information to the entire body about the foot and the body's relationship to space and movement.

The reflexognosist will follow four steps as part of a treatment protocol in their work.

Four Step Treatment Protocol
1. **Evaluation**
2. **Application**
3. **Assess Outcome**
4. **Re-evaluate**

Inspecting the Foot

For the professional reflexognosist there are many things to look for when inspecting the foot before beginning a session. First, if the client complains of foot pain, ask which foot gives the most trouble. Then examine the other foot, so you know more what a 'normal' foot is for the client. Foot assessment involves the following ten steps:

1. **Biomechanics/gait analysis.** Assess subtalar deviation and determine stress factors in muscle and skeletal framework. Observe how the client walks. Is there subtalar deviation to varus or valgus? A heavy heel strike or balanced 'toe off' (see page 106) to the hallux? Can the client balance on one foot at a time? Much of this can be confirmed with a prodotract.

2. **Shoes.** Notice the client's shoes. Have they been stretched to overrun the sole? What is the heel wearing pattern? The toe wearing pattern? Measure the client's foot, not just spacing, for proper shoe size *after* the treatment. The intrinsic muscles have relaxed and this will give the proper measurement. One exception to this is the possibility of edema around the foot or

ankle that may be made worse by hot weather. In this case the size of the foot will reduce during the session. This needs to be taken into consideration.

3. **Orthotics.** Does the client use arch supports and if so, how long have the orthotics been worn? They will need to be re-evaluated by their podiatrist as shifts in the feet occur with the application of reflexognosy.

4. **Color.** The foot changes color in weight-bearing and non-weight-bearing positions. Normally it takes a few seconds for the color to change when there is a change in position. If the foot is a light pink when elevated, but becomes very red when lowered, there may be a vascular disturbance or arterial insufficiency. The practitioner can also note disturbance in temperature by touch. A healthy blood flow is directly related to good health. This is an important evaluation.

5. **Swelling.** Check for unilateral or bilateral swelling. Unilateral swelling is usually due to an injury. Bilateral swelling may be evidence of circulation problems including the lymph or pelvic obstructions affecting venous return.

6. **Abnormalities.** Notice any pathologies or abnormalities of the foot. Investigate the foot for any corns or calluses—the foot being worn in a certain way. Note rashes, blisters, hammer toes, lacerations or varicose veins. Ascertain if

there has been any foot surgeries. Assess joint articulations and note restricted joint movement.

7. **Toes.** The toes should appear straight, flat and in proportion to each other and be similar to the other foot. Note variations from normalcy. If the toes do not perform their role properly additional energy is required to perform the complex task of movement.

8. **Peripheral vascular circulation.** How is the client's circulation? Is it slow and sluggish or normal? A quick test is to *gently* squeeze the hallux and count how long it takes for full color to return to the toe: Two seconds is considered normal. In the elderly, those who have had cardio-vascular disturbance, or those with diabetes, it may be found that they have a peripheral vascular return reading of 6-10 seconds, so be careful with your pressure when you squeeze the toe. Reflexognosy will assist peripheral vascular return. This is one of the major strengths of this discipline.

9. **Pain.** Ascertain if there is any pain when standing or walking and identify the exact location. Note pain anywhere in the body, not just in the feet.

10. **Common Foot Pathologies.** There are many pathologies that affect the feet. Most require treatment by a podiatrist. The most common symptoms are:

a) **Athlete's Foot** - also called tinea, is a highly contagious skin condition. Working on a person with tinea is contraindicated. The trend to work the area with the practitioner wearing gloves is not recommended due to the possibility of spreading the fungus to other locations on the client's foot. Do not work on the foot until the condition is cleared. A podiatrist or qualified reflexognosist will advise treatment.

b) **Bunion** - [hallux valgus] a tendon abducts [pulls] the hallux toward the other toes. Gentle movements of plantar flexion, dorsiflexion, abduction and adduction will be of assistance in reducing pain and may prove to be of value in slowing the deformity.

c) **Tailor's bunion** - is a small bunion on the lateral side of the foot affecting the 5th digit. Management is the same as for the hallux valgus.

d) **Calluses** - these are formed by dry pressure and friction. Most common sites for calluses are at the heads of the metatarsals, or the medial side of the hallux.

e) **Claw toe** - the *distal* phalanx is bent causing the toe to draw up. Contraction of the distal phalanx can be attributed to

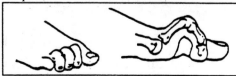

muscular tension in the foot and leg.

f) **Corns** - soft corns are most often found between the toes. They are soft due to the moisture between the toes. Hard corns are usually found on the dorsum of the toes in areas of excessive pressure. Both kinds of corns may be tender to direct pressure and require podiatric treatment.

g) **Hammer toe** - the *proximal* phalanx is bent causing the toe to draw up. This occurs because of muscle tension in the foot and leg.

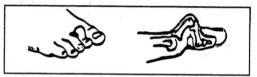

h) **Ingrown toenail** - a nail that is growing into the side of the toe. It is commonly found on the hallux and is a very painful condition requiring podiatric treatment.

i) **Neuroma** - is a tumor composed of nerve cells. The tumor is formed because of irritation to the nerve sheath. A neuroma is frequently found between the 3rd and 4th metatarsal heads. It can cause numbness and cramping and requires podiatric assistance.

j) **Plantar Fasciitis** - inflammation of the plantar fascia. Great care must be taken as the pain can be exacerbated by inappropriate touch. Oftentimes the primary cause of the problem is in the leg. The belly of the Flexor Digitorum Longus tightens and no longer elongates or flexes normally. The belly of the muscle must be released to increase circulation. Once circulation is increased through relaxation of the soft tissue and joint activation reducing inflammation and pain, healing can take place. Podiatric assistance is recommended if inflammation and pain continue.

k) **Plantar warts** - These are warts growing on the bottom [plantar surface)] of the foot. They are highly contagious and again, a podiatric referral is warranted.

l) **Gout** - the medial aspect of the first metatarsal head is a common site for gout which is caused by the deposit of urate crystals. Extreme pain may be felt by the client. Referral to a wholistically trained health care professional in the field of nutrition for dietary advice is suggested.

Practitioner Tactile Awareness

In looking at the foot as a foot in a wholisitic manner one must move beyond anatomy and physiology and examine the foot from all perspectives. This includes what the practitioner observes upon palpation.

Performing reflexognosy is not simply picking up a foot and leg and working them. The physical action of applying pressure to an area is simple—anyone can do it. But if reflexognosists are going to call themselves professionals, or make claims about reflexognosy, and if a person is going to charge

for services, then there must be an understanding of what is being felt. It takes time to learn the art of reflexognosy. The development of specific skills and their application is a lengthy process. For instance, anyone can learn to give a hypodermic injection in a few minutes, but to understand what happens physiologically to the tissue, the chemical reaction the drug is expected to produce and why, what reaction the patient may experience, etc. takes a nurse years of study. Receiving the best education available and keeping it current is important for reflexognosists. This requires time. It is the professional and responsible way to practice the art and enables the practitioner to deliver the finest and most up-to-date service.

Tactile awareness is very important to the reflexognosist as many things may be felt while touching and palpating the client's foot. The relaxed, flexible foot, one with good tone, makes balanced contact with the ground through locomotion and provides a firm support for the structure above. This produces an environment in which the foot is capable of handling whatever changes are encountered through movement.

Every client who presents to a reflexognosist poses a 'picture'. This picture is not one dimensional, but is as many faceted as the person. All the signs are expressed in various forms on the feet.

To the reflexognosist, the foot is an indicator of what is 'going on' with the *whole* person, the seen and the unseen. In previous eras the practitioner or physician was an astute and patient observer of the client—in many cases this is a lost art today. Reflexognosists are aided in observing the client by their knowledge of biomechanics and are encouraged, by their training, to incorporate every aspect of the client's being to assist in achieving a constructive outcome.

Generally, a hard, tense muscle is a stressed or strained muscle. By checking such things as ankle rotation one can feel a sense of whether or not the entire foot is flexible or stiff, relaxed or stressed. This can be an indicator of the condition for the entire body.

Beyond this basic feeling of the tissue, the tissue can take on different characteristics. Tissue that feels tight, taut, and painful is tissue under stress. If it is only stressed, moving the foot in different directions will usually relax the tissue and the stress will dissipate. First the tissue is relaxed by applying techniques, then the area is palpated again. If the sensitivity is gone or lessened it was probably due to the muscle being under strain. Pathological congestion, on the other hand, will be experienced as tense tissue which, when pressed, stays slightly depressed.

As pressure is applied over the foot, different sensations will be felt by the practitioner. In some literature 'little grains of sand' or 'crystals of sugar-like substances' are described as being felt. This is a lay attempt at describing a collection of debris that may feel like this. Adhesions or calcification that has formed between the layers of muscle, fascia or connective tissue is a more accurate and professional description of what is palpated.

Sometimes a hard lump on the plantar surface will be felt that is about the size of a pea. It will usually be sensitive and may be bilateral. This can be an accessory sesamoid. While two sesamoids are commonly found on the head of the first metatarsal, there are many sites for accessory sesamoids and nothing is wrong in the foot nor is it a sensitive reflex. This is why it is essential that a full and clear understanding of the possible anatomy be learned as part of training in reflexognosy.

Tactile experiences will differ between practitioners, frequently from client to client with the same practitioner and definitely within the same foot. Tactile awareness is acquired over time and comes with

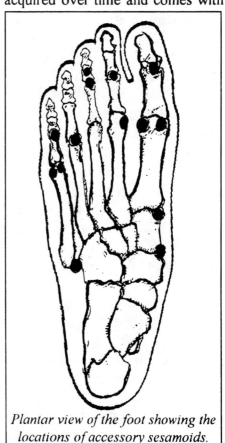

Plantar view of the foot showing the locations of accessory sesamoids.

experience. Bony landmarks should be studied, linking them together and obtaining a clear mental image of the skeletal layout beneath the area being palpated. Anatomy will become clearer and more understandable as the hands become more sensitive to what lies below the skin. Tactile awareness gives the practicioner remarkable insights into the condition of the feet that are presented.

What Does the Client Feel?

The practitioner must have the knowledge to assess the foot in 'real' terms. The reflexognosist will evaluate the foot and develop a treatment plan based on the findings. One indicator is the pain or amount of sensitivity the client feels. Tenderness can be misleading as it may indicate local or reflex problems in acute or chronic dysfunction. Its presence should be noted and this should lead to further palpation and observations with an open mind. The following is an overview as to why and where pain may be felt during a session. The reader will note there is no reference to organ congestion or dysfunction. It is the opinion of the authors that pain felt in the foot as a direct result of palpation usually has its cause in the foot. Appropriate palpation of the foot will reduce this discomfort. Reflexognosy will produce changes to the entire body but first the foot must be assessed and then proper techniques applied. Once the foot is able to perform its tasks correctly there will be a reduction in stress on the entire body.

Pain is multi-dimensional. It can be attributed to many possibilities depending on location. Pain is a function of the subtle energy body. It is invisible, yet it is felt at the physical level. Pain acts as a bridge between the physical (cellular) body and the subtle energy bodies. It can also be related to suppressed emotional disturbances. Therefore the reflexognosist will not jump to any hasty conclusions. Judgment must be withheld until further investigative work on the foot is performed and a detailed client history is taken.

In review, the following is a list of physical reasons why the client may experience sensitivity as the reflexognosist works over the foot.

1. Stressed tissue/lesions

2. Origins or insertions of muscles and tendons

3. Calcification formed between the layers of the intrinsic muscles of the foot

4. Neuroma

5. Malalignment of the bones in the foot

6. Heel spur

7. Sesamoid bones sensitivity

8. Tuberosity of the 5th metatarsal stressed by tendon attachments

9. Tightness of the fascia

10. Scar tissue and/or adhesions of the tissue

11. Injury to the bones and joints

12. Foreign objects embedded in the foot

13. Poor biomechanics causing stress factors

14. Corns, calluses and bunions

15. Heads of the metatarsophalangeal joints inflamed due to poor mechanics

16. Poorly fitting shoes

17. Inflammation

Note the absence of tender reflexes being mentioned. Dealing with anatomy and physiology there are any number of reasons for pain. Once the reason is ascertained the practitioner will access what body cavity would be affected as each part of the foot has a key stress area.

Foot Pain: Its Locations and Possible Reasons	
Location	**Professional Rationale**
General Pain	Bones not aligned
Pain between metatarsals-- dorsal aspect	Tight interosseus and or lumbrical muscles due to footwear, locomotion, bones malaligned
Pain plantar/anterior aspect of calcaneus	Heel spur—plantar fasciitis— Achilles tendonitis—contracted triceps surae, spur, deviation in subtalar joint.
Pain over 1st metatarsophalangeal joint	Bunion—inflammation of bursal sac due to irritation— Flexor tendon aggravated as it passes through the sesamoids
Pain over the tuberosity of the 5th metatarsal	Insertion points of peroneus muscle group—poor mechanics of foot at dorsiflexion—excessive supination due to subtalar varus
Knotted feeling along midline (in the soft tissue)	Lesion formed due to mechanics—tightness of the foot fascia due to poor development of intrinsic muscles—pronated foot subtalar valgus
Transversely across heads of metatarsophalangeal joints	Sensitive due to complex ligaments and muscle attachments —Complex field of tendons—Corns—Metatarsalgia
Pain on palpation of the extensor digitorum brevis	This muscle sits in the ditch created by the cuboid, sitting slightly behind the 5th metatarsal at its tuberosity. It is a delicate intrinsic muscle of the foot and performs complex tasks. Stress within this muscle will make it very tender. If the cuboid is not seated correctly this muscle will have an edematous feel to it.
Pain along medial border of the foot	This part of the foot houses several intrinsic muscles as well as several key jointed areas of the foot. Additionally major ligaments that assist in the formation of arches are housed here. A pronated foot will add problems to this area.
Lateral anterior aspect of ankle—bony areas or the extensor digitorum brevis sitting at the base of the 4th & 5th metatarsals affecting the cuboid	This section of the foot is under quite a degree of stress with every step we take. The tendons are an extension of the extrinsic muscles located in this area encased by the retinaculum. Deviation from normalcy in the gait patterns will limit the activity of the extrinsic muscles, stressing the tendons. This is a key reason for palpation in this area.
Pain around the lateral ankle	Due to a greater range of motion on the lateral side of the foot than the medial, more mechanical movement is felt. Deviation from normalcy will stress the intrinsic anatomy, muscles, tendons, and ligaments producing discomfort.

Chart 3

Foot Pain: Its Locations and Possible Reasons	
Location	**Professional Rationale**
Pain in the toes	An inflammation of the nerve between the 3rd and 4th metatarsal bones. The head of one metatarsal is pressing against another or pressing against a phalanx catching the nerve in between areas. When due to mechanical faults in the foot causing the toes to grip the nerve between the metatarsals, a condition known as **Morton's neuroma** may develop.
Pain on posterior calcaneus	Achilles tendinitis or retrocalcaneal bursitis
Sensitivity diagonally across the foot from the tuberosity of the 5th metatarsal to the head of the 1st metatarsal	Tenderness along the peroneus longus
Pain on posterior calcaneus (with bony prominence lateral to tendon)	'Pump bump' which is often associated with shoes—usually the shoes are too short.

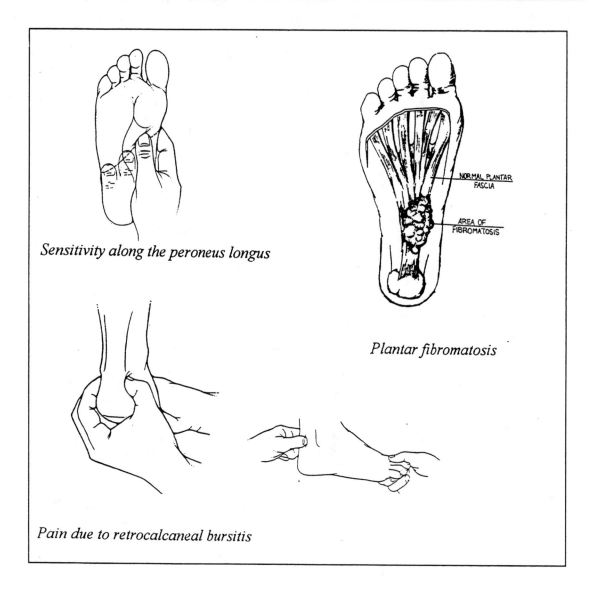

Sensitivity along the peroneus longus

NORMAL PLANTAR FASCIA

AREA OF FIBROMATOSIS

Plantar fibromatosis

Pain due to retrocalcaneal bursitis

Touch: the Sensual Aspects of Reflexognosy

In order to complete the investigation of the foot as a foot, we must examine the often overlooked sensual aspect. Unfortunately in our Freudian society sensuality is often confused with sexuality. The proper definition for sensual is sensory. To compound the confusion the tactile stimulation of touch itself carries many different meanings as does the intent of the practitioner. Compassionate touch is an important component of reflexognosy and it in itself is a powerful effective and non-invasive form of therapy. Touch conveys a welcome emotional message. It overcomes the feeling of isolation and provides a bridge of trust that allows people to communicate their fears.

Traditional Western medicine has ignored this aspect of human need. The art of touching the leg and foot in reflexognosy sets the stage for change, but technique can never make change happen, that lies with the client. The practitioner is a facilitator, not a healer. Healing takes place from within the client. It may be assisted by the practitioner, but not come from the practitioner.

Touch is vital to everyone's health, at any age, and is one of the body's basic needs. Touch is just as important as food and water. Centuries ago a group of orphans were deprived of touch and every one of them died, even though they had food and water. This same experiment, producing similar results, has often been repeated in this century using animals.[1] Touching is a way of showing care; that the person being touched is acceptable. A lack of touch brings social isolation which is common with many age groups within our society, especially the elderly. One aspect of social isolation is depression, reduced self-esteem and loneliness. Reflexognosy is one way of being touched in a non-threatening way because no clothes, except footwear, need to be removed. Reflexognosy is an 'acceptable' way of giving the body the sensual experiences it needs. Touch is only one of the vehicles reflexognosists utilize in giving rise to the body's own natural healing potential.

In addition, proper touch is relaxing. Relaxing all the tissue of the feet and legs with our hands will create a physiological response in the body. It will allow the person to walk differently and take strain off the body. The complexity of the foot leads us away from the notion that pressing a point immediately infers organs dysfunction. Other options to consider include:

1. Structure

2. Pathology

3. Replication

Anatomy and physiology of the body is, for the most part, the same for each individual. Likewise, the study of anatomy and physiology is similar with most disciplines, however, the theory and application in reflexognosy is different than other professions. In our case it consists of the *interconnection* between:

- the systems of the body and

their functions

- the foot as a structure [i.e., nerves, tissues, biomechanics]

- the map of the reflexes in the feet [i.e., reflexes as they are thought to exist and anatomically reflected on the feet]

- pathology in relation to the systems and

- how all of the above are affected by stimulation of the feet through pressure and touch.

The study of reflexognosy includes:

- hands-on application

- palpation of landmarks of the feet

- identification and reflexing of reflexes and other tissue in relation to the theory of the body being replicated on the feet.

The physical mechanisms through which reflexognosy works includes, but is not limited to:

- the nervous systems

- subtle energy systems

- circulatory and lymphatic systems

- sensory stimulation

- biomechanics

- zones

- touch

- the relaxation response.

These differences are what makes reflexognosy unique and a separate discipline from other professions.

Though not usually referred to as an organ, the foot is a complex organ adapted to the performance of specific functions. It has a great relevance to the rest of the body. Reflexognosists acknowledge this contribution and use their discipline as a 'gateway to healing' through the non-invasive treatment of the feet. In the next chapter we shall focus on the foot as an organ through the investigation of its biomechanical function.

---

[1] Montague, Ashley. *Touching: The Human Significance of the Skin*, 3rd Edition. Harper & Row, New York, 1971.

Chapter 9

Biomechanics & Reflexognosy

"Feet that are not optimally balanced are not giving you the support you need. In fact, feet which have lost their optimal structure, or have failed to adequately develop, are enemies to contend with at each step."

—Rick James

Bio means life, and mechanics means movement. Biomechanics of the leg and foot is the study of the locomotion or the mechanical movement of the body part. The biomechanical function of the leg and the foot, specifically focuses on assessing walking. The foot moves the body through locomotion. In walking, circulation is assisted, lymphatic flow is promoted, and activity through the central nervous system is stimulated. The sensory nervous system is sent messages through the foot touching the ground. The autonomic nerve ganglia is stimulated by sending messages of activity through the brain back down the spinal column to the messengers outside the spinal column to the autonomic nervous system which in turn sends the messages to the organs. Because of this important link the professional reflexognosist needs to understand the feet—their importance, and the importance of biome-

chanics and why this knowledge is inseparable from reflexognosy. Research shows that under every callus, corn, flat or misaligned foot is a stressed structure.

Foot Curve

An impression of a foot curve provides the podiatrist with an analysis of how the foot is moving during locomotion and if it is balancing the body correctly. To the reflexognosist it can indicate the different body cavities which are being stimulated or stressed by ineffective mechanics.

Not only in the simple act of walking is activity enacted by the foot and leg, but there is an unconscious participation of most of the muscles, organs, and tissues of the body in some way. Walking employs about two-thirds of the muscles of the body. The trunk muscles contract to hold the body upright as the leg moves, the arms swing forward and back involving the shoulder and hip flexors and the wrist extensors. In breathing, the diaphragm, abdominal muscles, and the muscles of the ribs expand the chest and lungs. Fuel and oxygen for the muscle action is brought by the arteries of the circulatory system which involves the heart, lungs, and nerves. In turn, waste products are carried away and filtered through the organs and glands. The foot acts not only as a way to move the body, but also as a sense organ. The nerves carry the stimuli for contraction to the muscles and the sense of position to the central nervous system. All this activity with each step!

With a normal foot curve the person locomotes and does not adversely stress other parts of the body. However, the normal foot curve is found in a low percentage of the population. In a normal step, the first point of contact with the ground is the heel—slightly to the lateral aspect. The weight is then carried along the outer border of the foot and across the ball to the great toe. At no point along this movement is the total foot flat on the ground. In a normal step there is a dynamic flow of energy from the heel out through the hallux.

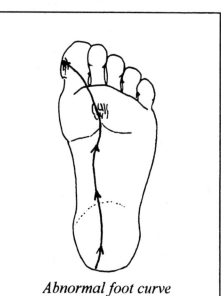

Abnormal foot curve

The incorrect foot curve places stress on the foot and sets up restriction in the anatomy of the foot. This restriction contributes to callus formation, corns and may be attributed to the development of bunions. Additionally the somatically replicated stress placed on the aligned body cavities during the locomotive phase must be considered.

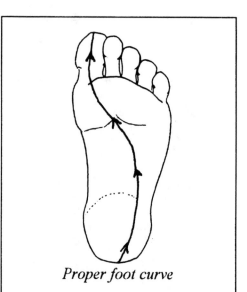

Proper foot curve

The correct foot curve will be balanced and cover the entire foot. The heel strike will be slightly to the lateral side and the 'toe off' will be felt through the center of the hallux. This indicates a foot that when locomoting is supinating—the normal gait pattern.

From a reflexognosy point of view, the normal foot curve reveals something dramatic. Following reflexognosy concepts, every time the foot moves through a range of locomotion the body mechanics are in harmony. As the foot starts to unload there is a balanced energy release, forward and back throughout the system. In a balanced foot curve the client is moving harmoniously with physical stress factors minimized.

The location of corns and calluses are very important to professional reflexognosists in the context of foot curve. They are due to pressure and friction as previously mentioned. If a reflexognosist finds signs of calluses, corns, bunions, and problems in the joints of the feet they will assess the foot curve. The foot curve provides accurate biomechanical feedback. These abnormalities indicate where the problems start, which in turn produces pressure or a lack of pressure on areas of the foot and may affect a somatically replicated part of the body. If you rectify the deviation then apply reflexognosy you will produce results. The treatment sequence, depending on the age and condition of the client, involves using relaxation techniques to relax the feet and legs, joint activation and assignment of daily range of movement exercises to strengthen muscles. If that does not correct the heel strike a referral to a podiatrist will be recommended.

When a person does not 'toe off' properly a callus may form somewhere along the medial side of the hallux. The podiatrist will look to skeletal problems in the spine, particularly in the neck because the major emphasis of weight, the anterior component of the body, is thrown forward jarring Cervical 1 to Cervical 7. The reflexognosist will draw the same conclusion by somatic replication.

The podiatrist would provide orthodics to produce a balanced foot curve. The reflexognosist would address those same areas using tactile means. Both professionals acknowledge that the rest of the body is affected by foot function. Both in their own fashion, attempt to remove the pressure, pain, or congestion and discomfort in the foot which is affecting the body.

Movements of the Foot

Reflexognosists are familiar with the following basic anatomical terminology in relation to movement of the feet. There are three paired movements of the feet. These include inversion and its opposite movement eversion, plantar flexion/dorsiflexion and abduction/adduction. These movements combine to perform the tri-plane action of either pronation or supination. The first two paired movements of abduction and adduction are single static biomechanical functions and not part of locomotion.

1. **Abduction.** Abduction means the foot or part of the body turns away from the mid-line. This includes any part of the foot as well as the whole foot.

2. **Adduction.** Adduction is moving toward the mid-line.

3. **Inversion.** Inversion occurs when the plantar surface of the foot actually turns toward the midline of the body. With inversion, the sole of the foot is tilted up more to face the midline of the body during the static stance. Inversion

shows on the soles of shoes as a wearing down on the lateral side.

4. **Eversion.** Eversion is the opposite of inversion. With eversion the plantar aspect of the foot is turned or tilted away from the midline. In this case shoes will wear on the medial side.

5. **Plantar flexion.** Plantar flexion is the foot and/or toes moving toward the ground (e.g. when a dancer points the toes).

6. **Dorsiflexion.** Dorsiflexion is the foot and/or toes moving up toward the body.

7. **Supination.** Supination is an action of movement and is not a static or stable stance. It is a tri-plane movement combining adduction, inversion, and plantar flexion.

8. **Pronation.** Pronation is the reverse of supination. Once again this is a tri-plane motion, but involves abduction, eversion and dorsiflexion.

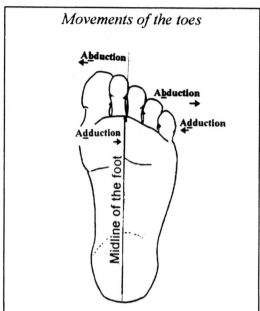

Movements of the toes

Toes work in relationship to the midline of the foot, not the midline of the body.

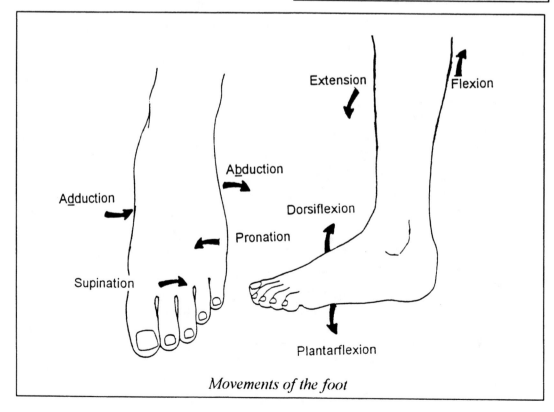

Movements of the foot

108

Valgus and Varus are terms used for either the positioning of the subtalar joint or the hallux.

9. **Valgus**. The valgus position is a specifically everted joint. The eversion will come through the hallux or the subtalar joint in the heel. Biomechanically, with a subtalar valgus, there is pressure to the hip and the organs that are housed within the pelvic cavity are affected. Lack of circulation to the legs can be a complaint with a subtalar valgus.

10. **Varus.** Varus is inversion of the part. Stress factors will be felt throughout the body. With subtalar varus, disturbance takes place to the lateral aspects of the body.

Other important terms

11. **Central point of gravity.** The central point of gravity means that as a person goes through a correct foot curve their central point of gravity will be at the central part of the pelvis. As a person pronates, the pelvis is thrown forward putting stress on the entire body and specifically on the pelvic cavity and the organs housed therein.

12. **Pes Cavus.** This condition is known as the high arched foot. The opposite condition is referred to as a flat foot—**pes plantus**.

13. **Bunions.** When a person has a bunion or hallux valgus, the rest of the foot compensates. Bones actually move to compensate for the pressure and the lack of supported structure within the medial sagittal plane or at the head of the metatarsophalangeal joint of the hallux.

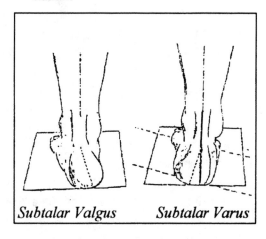

Subtalar Valgus   *Subtalar Varus*

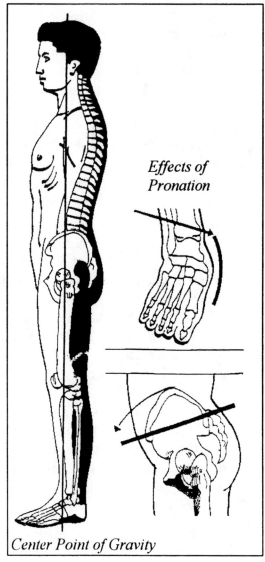

Effects of Pronation

Center Point of Gravity

Biomechanics and Physical Energy

As previously stated, on the physical level, there are two types of energy transfer occurring during walking—an exchange between potential and kinetic energy, and the transfer of energy between one limb segment and another. As well as the vertical motion of the trunk, there are other exchanges between potential and kinetic energy in the twisting of the shoulder girdle and pelvis in an opposite direction. Power is the rate at which energy is generated or absorbed in the process and is measured in watts. One of the remarkable features of normal gait is how energy is conserved by means of a number of optimizations. Abnormal gait patterns on the other hand may result in excessive fatigue. For instance, with pronation the central point of gravity is thrown off causing the pelvic region to tilt. This forms unrelenting stress and fatigue on the body with each step that is taken. The measurement by a podiatrist of energy consumption during walking can be an important element in scientific gait analysis assisting to form the treatment plan for the reflexognosist. When structural deviation from normalcy is rectified stress is relieved.

On the subtle energy level, the foot has a great deal to do with the body's energy exchange with the ground. It is a contact point for drawing in the electromagnetic energy of the earth. According to Tiller (1983), for most right-handed people and two-thirds of left-handed people the energy comes into the bottom of the left foot, up across the groin and out the right foot.[1]

Biomechanics and its Importance to Reflexognosy

The role of the medial aspect of the foot is shock absorption while the lateral side is the balancing agent of the foot. The complexity of the foot leads us away from the notion that pressing a point on the foot infers dysfunction in the organs of the body. In clinical practice, to claim that a point on the foot relates to the condition of an internal organ is to eliminate logic and critical thinking. A foot that is not functioning correctly can put other parts of the torso under stress, leading to health problems. A foot problem may lead to a damaging gait, which in turn puts the pelvis under stress. That could hinder the proper functioning of the bowel which results in constipation. Think for a moment about what areas should be stimulated everyday for health. One organ is the colon. The colon is stimulated through locomotion with our heel strike and its effect on the pelvic cavity. On 'toe off', with a balanced foot curve, there is improved oxygenation of the cranial cavity due to the circulatory and lymphatic system being stimulated via movement of the gastrocnemius. At the same time the somatically replicated areas of the major organs are lightly touched and gently stimulated. Everything to do with biomechanics of the foot and leg links with reflexognosy.

Body Cavity Link

As mentioned previously, structural deviation from normalcy in the feet will adversely affect the body. Reflexognosy hypothesizes and extends on the classical podiatric base that structural deviation from normalcy in the leg and foot affects the skeletal framework of the body by evaluating the changes to the organs and other body parts in an eclectic way. There are several interesting correlations between the feet and the body.

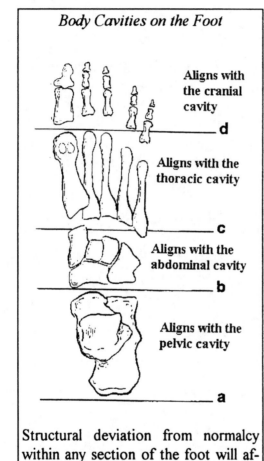

Body Cavities on the Foot

Aligns with the cranial cavity

d

Aligns with the thoracic cavity

c

Aligns with the abdominal cavity

b

Aligns with the pelvic cavity

a

Structural deviation from normalcy within any section of the foot will affect the associated body cavity directly and the entire body indirectly.

It is often overlooked by other health care professionals that structural deviation from normalcy in the feet will affect the skeletal framework. However, podiatrists have proven that deviation from normalcy in the rear foot will affect the sacroiliac joint and depending on the degree of deviation, will deter-

mine the inclusion of the thoracic and cranial structures. Reflexognosy links the structural deviation from normalcy in the feet and the function or dysfunction with the entire anatomy and physiology aligned to the cavity and beyond.

The more calluses, corns, or bunions; the more one excessively supinates or pronates; or presents with heavy calluses formation around the back of the heel; the moment one deviates from normalcy in gait patterns, all will detract from the proper biomechanical foot curve and present unwanted stress. From a reflexognosy point of view, areas are either not being stimulated or are being over stimulated. Regular reflexognosy sessions will be of benefit to overall health.

The paradigm shift to a wholistic approach is not great for the lay practitioner dealing with feet. The key transition is not to focus on one part, rather align thinking to the entire function of the body. This wholistic process will enable the professional practitioner to deal with the 'person' and their 'being'. The application of the discipline will enable the body's own innate intellect to interpret the touch and transmit through the body a change in function returning to a more normal structure, reducing stress factors. The internal healing environment that is naturally within is stimulated and assisted by reflexognosy. The credit for improvement of health belongs to the client's body and internal healing response to foot work.

In all medicine, deviation from normal structure occurs first, then the condition presents. Whether the aberration is a change in energy, emotional or spiritual, thinking or feelings, does not matter. What matters is a change in some process has occurred which is followed by a change in structure. Podiatry will talk about the affects of vibration from the foot and skeletal alignment during locomotion. In their philosophies, if jarring occurs at certain points particular problems will manifest. They may then prescribe orthotics to alter the biomechanics and ease the pain. Reflexognosists agree, but in their thought process the pressure will also affect the entire body not only skeletal alignment.

Gait analysis is observing the way the client walks to evaluate how the body moves. It involves checking the opposite side to see if the body is compensating. Through observation of deviations from normalcy in the foot and leg the reflexognosist will be able to assess which areas of the body are under strain and verify the finding through a comprehensive assessment procedure. The condition may not be present in the foot itself, but along a pathway. The first step toward change is assessing the structure of the foot and evaluate how it moves. Appraising the foundation of the body is as important as evaluating the foundation of a building in determining the entire structure's integrity.

Practical Application of Biomechanics

The ability of the practitioner in Reflexognosy to visually assess the locomotion pattern of the client is of paramount importance when determining the stress factors and where they may be occurring. For instance, if a client demonstrates a walking pattern of pronation the:

- medial side of the foot will be stressed
- a heavy callus may be detected at the head of the first metatarsal-phalangeal joint.

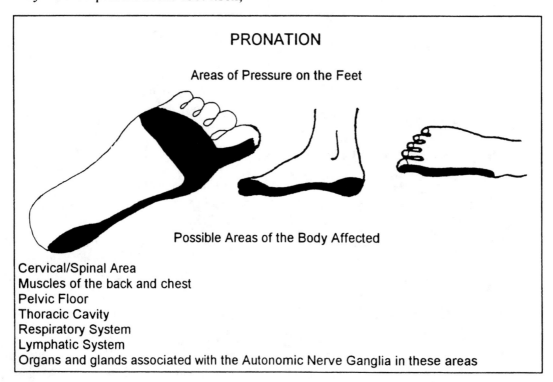

PRONATION

Areas of Pressure on the Feet

Possible Areas of the Body Affected

Cervical/Spinal Area
Muscles of the back and chest
Pelvic Floor
Thoracic Cavity
Respiratory System
Lymphatic System
Organs and glands associated with the Autonomic Nerve Ganglia in these areas

SUPINATION

Areas of Pressure on the Feet

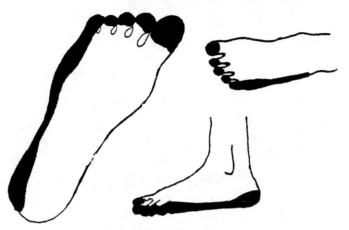

Possible Areas of the Body Affected

Tissue in the shoulder and arm area
Pelvic region - lateral area
Cranial Cavity
Lymphatic system

INVERSION

Areas of Pressure on the Feet

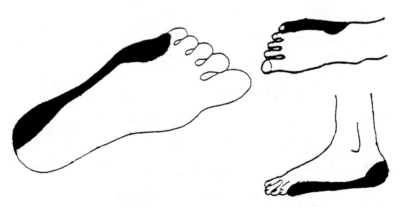

Possible Areas of the Body Affected

Tissue in the shoulder and arm area
Pelvic region - lateral area
Lymphatic System

EVERSION

Areas of Pressure on the Feet

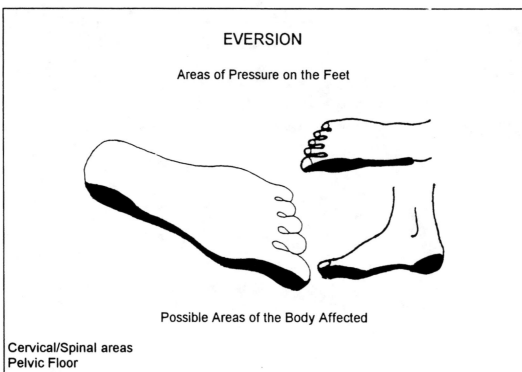

Possible Areas of the Body Affected

Cervical/Spinal areas
Pelvic Floor
Circulatory System
Lymphatic System
Organs and glands associated with the Autonomic Nerve Ganglia in these areas

DORSIFLEXION

Areas of Pressure on the Feet

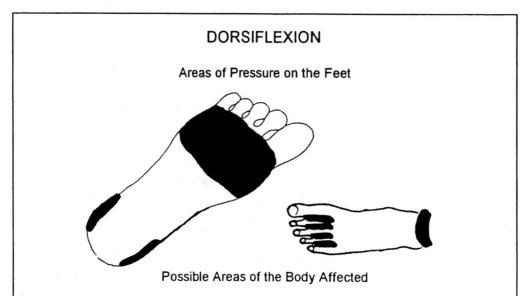

Possible Areas of the Body Affected

Pelvic Region
Thoracic Cavity
Lymphatic System
Organs and glands associated with the Autonomic Nerve Ganglia in these areas
Leg - as this movement may result in the tensing of the gastrocnemius both anteriorly and posteriorly, with the result being poor circulation and pressure put on the flow of lymph from the leg and foot areas.

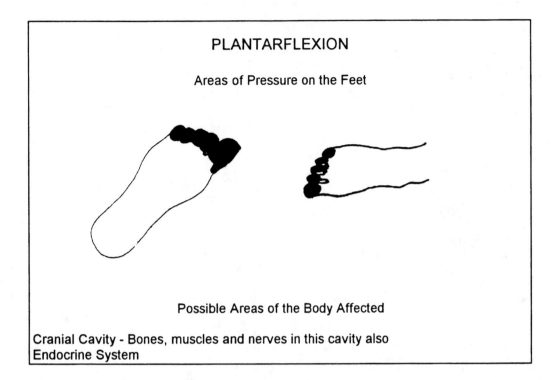

PLANTARFLEXION

Areas of Pressure on the Feet

Possible Areas of the Body Affected

Cranial Cavity - Bones, muscles and nerves in this cavity also
Endocrine System

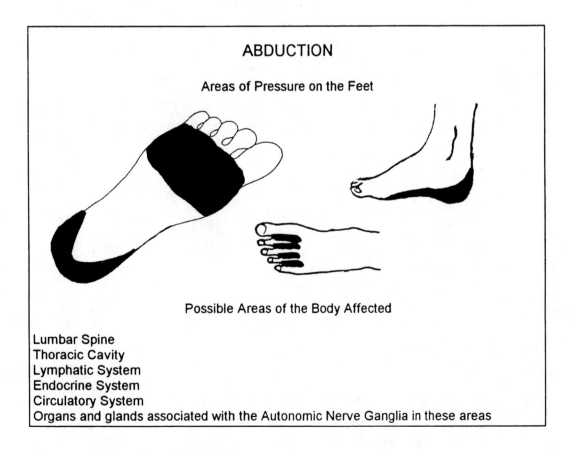

ABDUCTION

Areas of Pressure on the Feet

Possible Areas of the Body Affected

Lumbar Spine
Thoracic Cavity
Lymphatic System
Endocrine System
Circulatory System
Organs and glands associated with the Autonomic Nerve Ganglia in these areas

ADDUCTION

Areas of Pressure on the Feet

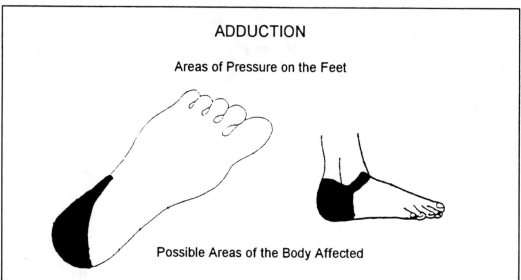

Possible Areas of the Body Affected

Pelvic Area
Organs and glands associated with the Autonomic Nerve Ganglia in this area
Lymphatic System
Leg and Knee - Pressure is strong in these two areas of the body resulting in a tightening of the gastrocnemius which could result in problems with blood flow or lymph flow to and from the feet. A force is also being exerted on the knee joint itself.

SUBTALAR VARUS

Areas of Pressure on the Feet

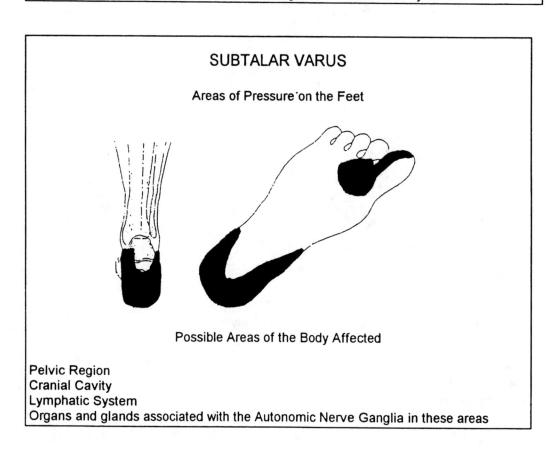

Possible Areas of the Body Affected

Pelvic Region
Cranial Cavity
Lymphatic System
Organs and glands associated with the Autonomic Nerve Ganglia in these areas

SUBTALAR VALGUS

Areas of Pressure on the Feet

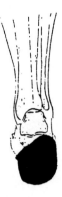 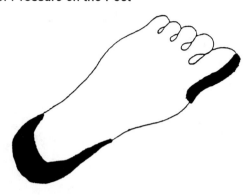

Possible Areas of the Body Affected

Lumbar Spinal Area
Cervical Spinal Area
Organs and glands associated with the Autonomic Nerve Ganglia in these areas including the endocrine system
Pressure may also result across the thoracic cavity

Conditions that are commonly seen would be:

- ankle edema

- knee pain

- sacroiliac joint pain

- elevated extensor digitorium brevis

- spinal pain which is usually emphasized in the lumbar region

Concentrating on the link between the foot and the body, indirect conditions that can develop from pronation include:

- general pelvic floor disturbances

- menstrual pain

- constipation

- hemorrhoids

- prostatitis

- bladder weakness

All of these conditions have a relationship to the way a person walks.

For the practitioners who wish to develop a wholistic understanding of the foot as an organ, management of soft tissue is also called for and will be explored in the next chapter.

---

[1] Tiller, William Ph.D. Audio Tape, *Energy Medicine 1* #6B, Edgar Cayce Foundation, Virginia Beach, Virginia, 1983.

Chapter 10

Soft Tissue Management & Reflexognosy

Foot comfort varies directly with foot function
—John Martin Hiss

The most important part of any physical structure is the foundation and for the body that foundation is the feet. Movement, blood circulation, lymphatics, and stimulation of all the nervous systems—all this activity generates from our feet! People literally die from the feet up. Medically speaking, when a patient is dying the feet are the first sign of approaching death. In turn, as experienced through reflexognosy, the body can heal from the stimuli provided to the feet.

Just as the masseur must know the muscles and the skeletal framework of the body to do massage, the reflexognosist must know biomechanics of the leg and foot as well as the structure of the foot. Everything to do with the foot and leg. Without locomotion the body goes nowhere, and without movement life stagnates and the body wastes away.

Periosteum

Understanding the soft tissue of the foot is an important part of, not only knowing the foot, but the total body as well. With the complexity of the anatomy of the foot it is little wonder that pain occurs. First and foremost, pain in the foot means dysfunction within the foot.

On the plantar aspect there are four layers of delicate muscles, each layer taking an enormous amount of stress as the body stands and moves. If the foot is mechanically sound it will perform like a well-oiled machine, if not then pain and discomfort is experienced. When the muscles are constantly forced to adapt to unnatural maneuvers they will succumb to pressure and become injured. Consideration must also be given to the complex linking of the tendons and ligaments, as they too will become painful and dysfunctional if forced to perform under pressure. One of the most overlooked but sensitive areas of the foot is the periosteum, the fine covering over the bone.

Periosteum is a specialized connective tissue covering all bones of the body. It consists of two layers.

The external layer is a network of dense connective tissue containing blood vessels. The deep layer is composed of more loosely arranged collagenous bundles with spindle-shaped connective tissue cells and a network of thin elastic fibers. Periosteum serves as a supporting structure for blood vessels nourishing bones and for attachment of muscles, tendons, and ligaments. Another function of the periosteum involves remodeling of the bone in the healing of fractures. Periosteum membrane is thick and markedly vascular over young bones but thinner and less vascular in later life. Bones that lose periosteum through injury or disease usually scale or die.

Periosteum and Reflexes

In 1944 Inman and Saunders mapped segmental innervation of the periosteum. By the 1950s German doctors Vogler and Krauss had detected pathological changes in the periosteum when palpitated. According to Dr. Ross Turchaninov, M. D. these changes have reflex characteristics in two ways:

1. Elimination of pain and delayed development of the degenerative process in the joints; as well as

2. Interrupting a vicious cycle which takes place between the affected inner organs and the reflex zones in the periosteum by restoring local metabolism and balancing relations between the inner organs [viscera] and the corresponding parts of the body [soma].[1]

"Reflex zones appear secondarily to the main disorder and are located either in the skin, connective tissue structures [fascia, aponeurosis], skeletal muscles or the periosteum. Reflex zones interconnect with one another when they are innervated by the same pair of spinal nerves. In the skin, reflex zones can be detected as areas of excessive dermoraphism, circulatory disorders, numbness, paraesthesia and cutaneous trigger points. In the connective tissue, the reflex zones are called connective tissue zones. They are represented by local edema, reactive points and fibrotic connections between skin and fascia. In the skeletal muscles, the reflex zones are seen as different types of hypertonic pathology [i.e. hypertonus, trigger points, myogelosis]. The reflex zones in the periosteum are represented either by local pain [i.e. periosteal trigger points] or by the changing structure of the periosteum. Such a change involves local thickening, roughness and condensation,"[2] writes Turchaninov.

In periostal massage, a specialty branch of medical massage, trigger points are located all over the body including in the hands and feet. Trigger points in the hands are found at the wrist and heads of the metacarpal bones while in the feet along the calcaneus (both lateral and medial), the lateral and medial malleous, mid shaft on the metatarsal bones, and on the tuberosity of the 5th metatarsal—all common sites associated with the reflex areas of other foot therapies. In these areas only a small part of the periosteum is accessible since it is covered by skin, or skin and a thin muscular layer. The periosteum may be very sensitive.

An extremely painful condition and one regularly overlooked by therapists working on the feet is periosteitis. In mild cases the condi-

120

tion may be activated by trauma to the actual foot itself or in serious cases of acute infection. The condition is characterized by tenderness and swelling of the bone affected. In more advanced cases fever and chills may be present.

It is important to stress that no one should attempt to treat a painful condition unless it has been adequately diagnosed by a physician or other qualified health care practitioner. Pain is a warning signal that must be respected. It is an indication that something may be seriously wrong and directs the reflexognosist to make a referral. Once the physician has cleared the client to receive reflexognosy, stimulation to the periosteum, because of its rich nerve and blood supply can cause changes in the area treated which often results in the relief of pain. However, deep penetrating palpation is never necessary. No therapy can be called useful if great pain is felt. Pain under all circumstances means dysfunction and injury. The foot is no different.

If deep, heavy palpation is applied to areas of the foot, pain may be felt. This is due to the sensitivity of the bone and the periosteum. The origin and insertion points of the intrinsic muscles are usually also quite painful if the foot is not:

1. handled correctly by the practitioner

2. supported by the practitioner and

3. an awareness of the areas where muscles are under the most stress is not considered by the practitioner.

A few examples are:

1. Origin at the calcaneus of the abductor hallucis brevis

2. Origin of the Flexor Digitorum Brevis and

3. Origin of the Abductor Digiti Quinti

Deep palpation to these areas with the foot in a dorsiflexed position will guarantee pain and discomfort for no other reason than the area is actually quite sensitive, made more so if the muscles are activated by the foot being placed in a dorsiflexed position.

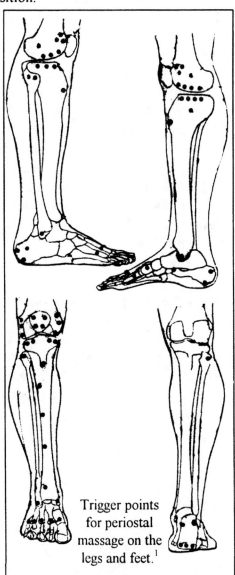

Trigger points for periostal massage on the legs and feet.[1]

Stanley Rosenberg writes in *Pain Relief with Osteomassage*, gentle stimulation of the nervous system through pressure to the periosteum, encourages the body to recognize the 'danger' or 'injury' is gone. The parasympathetic nervous system is activated and brings with it relaxation.

According to Dr. Ronald M. Lawrence, M.D. in the same book, there are approximately 120 osteopoints in the body. Light pressure is used to stimulate the nerves surrounding the bone. He claims it is enough to just feel, slightly, the surface of the hard part of the bone. Light touch facilitates sensing of the body's own feedback system. According to Lawrence, the client may experience a dull, aching sensation generated by either pressure which indicates the treatment is going to be effective. However, a sharp pain means the therapist is over stimulating the area. In this case, results will still be obtained but it is not wise to subject someone to such discomfort. Lawrence also contends, chronic problems respond to heavier pressure than do acute problems. The more acute the pain problem the less pressure is needed to control it.[3]

As with acupuncture the reflexognosist's intent is not to work on specific osteopoints or posteriosteum reflexes, except as they coincide with reflexognosy work on the feet.

Joint Activation

Soft tissue aside, another occurrence that impairs circulation to an area is an inflexible joint. An inflexible joint impairs circulation to its area. If the foot and joints are not optimally balanced the rest of the

body cannot be balanced because of poor biomechanics of the foot and leg. The way you walk, every step you take, every movement you make with the foot is going to effect the entire structure of the body, including organs, muscles and bones. Research has documented that biomechanics of the feet can be linked to illness. This means that the way we walk and the subluxation of bones in our feet affects our health immensely. Without the correction of subluxations, energy is impeded to a large degree. Joint activation assists in the relaxing and releasing of the soft tissue of the feet which allows ligaments to normalize the position of the bones for proper biomechanical function.

Understanding what is occurring in the underlying aspect of the foot which is causing stress and pressure, can be linked to joint pains throughout the body, the spine and to specific conditions that present. It must be repeated that reflexognosy deals with 'people', not disease or illness. Reflexognosists will understand the processes, but will focus on the person.

Introduction to Foot Function and the Work of Dr. John Martin Hiss

The foot and ankle are the focal points to which the total body weight is transmitted when walking. The heel and toes operate as shock absorbers and the joints are capable of adjustments necessary for balance. The effects of the bones in the feet 'being out of place' will be felt throughout the body. 'Bad feet, bad spine, bad health', is an easy way to remember the importance of the feet as the foundation of our physical structure. In addition, you cannot get the best results with reflexognosy if the delicate bones are not positioned correctly. With your hands it is easy to relax the foot and assist in the realigning of the foot, thereby unblocking energy and expediting the healing process. Reflexognosists *DO NOT* manipulate, they activate the joints by releasing the soft tissue.

Dr. John Martin Hiss, an osteopath, medical doctor, orthopedic surgeon and lecturer on functional foot disorders evaluated 300,000 feet in his career before writing *Functional Foot Disorders* in 1949. His son, also a medical doctor, wrote the introduction to each chapter of this classic. As an internist he believed the foot to be an integral part of the functioning of the body and implored his fellow physicians to consider the foot in general diagnostic procedures.[4]

The seven fundamental functions of the feet according to Hiss are to:[5]

1. Support and

2. Balance the body

3. Move it through locomotion

4. Adapt the body to changing positions

5. Distribute the weight of the body across the foot during walking

6. Transform potential energy into mechanical energy and

7. Contribute to the vitality of the entire organism.

Comfort, according to Hiss, varies directly with the functional ability of the foot. The common causes of functional foot disorders in Hiss' opinion are improper shoes and the sum total of slight injuries sustained by the feet over a lifetime.

Anatomically there is a great deal of tissue in the leg and foot to consider before performing joint activation. It is critical that the soft tissues [the muscles, tendons, ligaments and other tissue] be assessed and relaxed. In order to relax the muscles in the foot prior to joint activation one must start where they begin, in the leg. Although one is working with the joints, nerves are important also, especially around the cuboid. There is a close relationship between the cuboid tuberosity and the lateral plantar nerve. The posterior tibial nerve divides to form the medial plantar and lateral plantar nerves. In the region of the cuboid the lateral plantar divides into the superficial and deep branches. The nerves are separated from the cuboid by the thin quadratus plantar muscle. Any downward and inward rotation of the cuboid bone, if it be only 1/8 inch will cause an encroachment of the tuberosity upon the superficial trunk of the lateral plantar nerve. Simple pressure on the sole of the foot at this cuboid will cause severe pain, often with shooting pains into the 4th toe.

Anterior to the cuboid the medial aspect of the superficial portion of the lateral plantar nerve [which supplies the 4th toe and half of the 3rd and 5th toes] becomes more superficial as it passes around the muscle belly of that part of the flexor digitorum brevis that moves the 5th toe. This muscle is commonly in a state of contracture from general foot strain, and that portion that moves the 5th toe is in such close proximity to this nerve that pressure irritation is possible here also.

The superficial portion of the lateral plantar nerve supplies motor branches to the 4th plantar interosseus, the flexor digiti quinti brevis, and the opponens digiti quinti muscles. Mechanical irritation of the lateral plantar nerve can cause cramping in any one of these muscles. Lateral plantar nerve irritation from the rotated cuboid may cause pain, numbness, and hot and cold sensations in the 3rd, 4th and 5th toes. Gliding the cuboid back in place usually removes the pressure and provides immediate relief. This is achieved by selecting specialized techniques to the muscle group, moving away from the bone during the procedure. This is a complex procedure, far more than pressing points, finding sensitivity and inferring organ congestion.

Testing for normal foot function can be performed by reflexognosists to determine alignment of the feet.

- The arch may appear to be high or low

- The normal balanced foot will have perfect alignment

- An average range of function

- Be comfortable and pain free with ordinary usage.

However, there are a number of pathologies to be aware of. While a visual observation may indicate the above, in a problem known as 'Locked Joint', in spite of perfect alignment, there will be limited motion and the client will complain the foot is quite painful. Metatarsalgia is another common problem because of the failure of the foot to distribute weight across the metatarsal heads due to poor function in the rear foot. In addition loss of comfort and function may center around subluxations of first cuneiform and the cuboid. A further cause of pain and limited range of movement may come from the navicular.

The goal of joint activation is to restore foot function by overcoming joint tension, relieving muscle strain, and increasing range of motion. Joint activation is not a cure-all. The practitioner's intent is to bring the foot back to a stage within *compensatory limits* where it will be comfortable. Therefore, one is not necessarily trying for a 100% realignment of bones and tissue. The reflexognosist *never* forces any movement. That could do more harm than good, especially if the client's body, over the years, has learned to compensate for malaligned bones and other structural problems, and the joints have fused.

Joint activation is a highly specialized technique. It is the opinion of the authors that training should only be provided to practitioners who have a clear understanding of the anatomy of the foot. There are several things to keep in mind when performing joint activation techniques:

- The bones to be released

- The reason for moving them

- The direction and plane upon which one expects to effect correction.

Correction is achieved by work on the soft tissue. Manipulations are the domain of podiatrists

Bones of the Feet	Relationship to Body Cavity
Talus, Calcaneus	Pelvic
Navicular, Cuneiforms, and Cuboid	Abdominal
Metatarsals	Thoracic
Phalanges	Cranial

and chiropractors, not reflexognosists. One needs to be specific in their intent and remain within their professional boundaries.

Subluxations of the Feet and Their Relationship to Body Cavities

Subluxation of the various bones of the feet can be related to the four body cavities. When a bone is subluxed, pressure can be brought to bear on the corresponding body cavity. In performing joint activation one is assisting nature to normalize, not forcing anything. Joint activation is not a matter of force. Comprehensive joint activation techniques are included as part of a total reflexognosy treatment. In the words of Millicent Linden (1968) in reference to the body "A total working unit means that all parts are in minimum conflict or friction with each other." [6] The reflexognosist works to restore balance and reduce tension by working with the body in a natural way through joint activation.

Joint Activation Utilizing PNF

One of the techniques used in joint activation is PNF Stretching. PNF Stretching, or Proprioceptive Neuromuscular Facilitation, is a unique stretching technique that will quickly relax the muscles of the leg and foot. It is a type of muscular re-education that helps the muscles relax

and unfold. Proprioceptors are neurological sensory receptors located throughout the body and are found primarily in the soft tissue, although they are also located in and around joints. They provide information to the brain concerning the status of the tissue—its state of contraction, how much tension is in the muscle tissue, the angle of the joint, and how much pressure is on it. PNF stretching is a physical therapy technique that was developed in the 1940s and 50s. It was used to treat individuals with neurological impairment. Today PNF stretching is used in order to gain increased flexibility and improvement in physical performance in sports training and sports massage. PNF stretching is the safest and most effective type of passive/active muscle stretch to achieve the results needed in a reflexognosy session.

PNF stretching relaxes the musculature in the leg and foot prior to a Reflexognosy session and joint activation procedures. PNF enables the practitioner to:

1. Assess range of movement [ROM)]of the foot and leg

2. Increase flexibility to intrinsic and extrinsic muscles

3. Improve circulation to the foot

4. Determine improvement in ROM of relevant joints

125

5. Utilize tactile sensitivity

6. Utilize the techniques as part of the evaluation process.

7. Work within safety parameters.

There are four stages in the application of PNF stretches:

1. Massage the leg and foot

2. Bring the part to neutral then contract—the muscle group is contracted using resistance. With pressure the client pushes against the reflexognosist's hand which is pushing in the opposite direction. This position is held for 10 seconds.

3. Relax for 5 seconds. To relax, the practitioner can flex the ankle several times checking for ROM.

4. Next, take the part to full resistance with the client offering no resistance.

Repeat steps 1-4 as often as necessary assessing effectiveness each time then move on to another muscle group.

There are six stretches essential to reflexognosy. The stretches work with the natural movement of the foot:

- plantar flexion

- dorsiflexion

- inversion

- eversion

- plantar flexion of the digits

- dorsiflexion of the digits

Resistance is offered in the opposing direction by the practitioner. Each

stretch is held for ten seconds, then released and allowed to relax for an additional few seconds before moving on to the next stretch. PNF stretching adds less than two minutes per foot to a session but promotes a more constructive outcome to the work.

A muscle is most relaxed, and may be more effectively stretched, immediately after isometric contraction. The relaxation lasts for about ten seconds, which is a safe time for a stretch. All these movements are performed as the reflexognosist is pushing in the opposite direction. It is necessary the client rest between each stretch. Stretches can be performed once for each of the six directions or as many times as it is felt necessary to increase the range of motion and relax muscles in the leg and foot. Muscles will respond favorably to stretch if 'warmed up' by soft tissue techniques before beginning these stretches. Select a range of techniques to provide warming to the area as a preliminary to PNF.

PNF is recognized as the safest and most effective type of muscle stretch as the client plays the active role by providing resistance and may reduce resistance if pain occurs. PNF stretching can be used for either prevention, correction, and or rehabilitation of the foot and leg muscles. The practitioner can provide the power to perform the stretch where there is muscle dysfunction or injury. In this case the client is passive. All passive stretches involve the reflexognosist moving the joint as far as the abnormally contracted muscle fibers will allow. The client contracts muscles to the stretch against resistance. Muscles are isometrically contracted for five seconds. The client then relaxes for five seconds. This procedure can be repeated until movement is obtained.

End-feel is the sensation of resistance which occurs during a passive stretch when the muscle has reached its end range of movement. Tactile sensitivity should enable the reflexognosist to perceive this resistance. For safety and comfort End-feel should never be exceeded in PNF stretching.

The reflexognosist will consider the action of the muscles of the leg as they are vital to foot movement. If the foot is biomechanically unsound, due to tightness of the muscles in the leg, it will be more difficult to obtain optimal results with reflexognosy. The trained reflexognosist will blend several professional techniques that will evaluate the position of the joints and bones and apply suitable correcting techniques. The inclusion of PNF stretching in a reflexognosy session has been found to produce dynamic results and is essential to perform before joint activation.

Often a painful site on the foot will completely disappear once PNF stretches have been performed. This tends to challenge the theory that a painful site indicates organ or gland dysfunction, and confirms that the pain in the foot is related to the foot itself.

Before joint activation it is critical to relax the fascia in the ankle and release the tension in the tendons. This results in the ability to assess tendons, ligaments and bone structure before activation because of bony extosis.

The number one cause of foot disorders according to Dr. Hiss is the shoes we wear. Dr. Simon Wikler DPM, speaking in front of a group of reflexologists in Toronto in 1990, agreed when he said, "Today orthotics and cosmetic surgeries are quick fixes for foot problems. They ignore what our shoes do to our feet, postures, and total health."[7] It is to the topic of foot wear and Wikler's views on this subject we shall now turn.

---

[1] Turchaninov, Ross. "Periostal Massage", *Massage & Bodywork*, June/July 1999, pg 26-36

[2] Ibid, pg. 27.

[3] Lawrence, Ronald and Stanley Rosenberg. *Pain Relief with Osteomassage*, Woodbridge Press, Santa Barbara CA 1982, pg. 79-80.

[4] Hiss, John Martin, *Functional Foot Disorders*, pg. X, intro

[5] Hiss pg.183-186

[6] Linden, Millicent. *Stretch for Life*, Information Incorporated, New York, 1968 pg. 15.

[7] Wikler, Simon. "A Guide to Foot Assessment for Reflexologists", *RAC/CNAR Conference Report*, 1990, pg 36.

Chapter 11

Assessment, Exercise & Footwear

Do not waste time trying to find the perfect shoe. There are none!
— **Simon Wikler**

'Feet, fabulous feet'. But when they are sick you feel bad all over. Therefore, it is essential to take care of these often overlooked parts of the anatomy and pamper them as the truly powerful health aids they are. They are going to effect your body with every step you take.

According to a study of 356 women conducted by the American Orthopaedic Foot and Ankle Society 88% of women wear shoes that are too small for their feet. This results in 80% of women suffering foot pain. The study also revealed 76% have deformities—hammertoes, bunions, etc. It cannot be emphasized enough that correct footwear influences health. Taking into consideration the movements previously referred to, footwear must be supportive and comfortable, allowing your feet to move during locomotion unrestricted.

The tissue of the normal foot is concerned with the very specialized function of locomotion. Aside from accidents, foot disorders of whatever kind, come from requiring the tissues

of the foot, or parts of the body vitally connected with the foot, or those participating in foot function, to continually function in a way different from that which determines their correct structure. Structural deviation from normalcy allows an abnormal situation to develop producing physiological change. Corns, blisters, calluses, and malaligned toes are examples of alteration in structure resulting from a forced modification in function by way of strain or pressure, or when the foot attempts to function normally in an ill-shaped or ill-fitted shoe. The continuous existence of a healthy foot depends upon normal foot functioning; the repair of an ailing foot depends upon whether the tissues of the foot are permitted to engage in their "proper mode of activity".

These are the thoughts of American podiatrist, Dr. Simon Wikler. He recognized that when the body is thrown anteriorly [forward] the shock absorption capacity of the foot is out of balance. During locomotion, if the shock of the foot's impact as it touches the ground is not absorbed, the body naturally wants to move forward to balance itself from the jarring. Wikler said the anterior plane of the body, comes straight down through the front part of the body and across the forefoot. If anything is disturbed in the anterior plane the body throws itself forward, and when the body throws itself forward stress in the frontal part of the body is the result. This pressure, Wikler concluded, was a contributing factor in heart disease and breast cancers. He recognized this connection in the 1950s!

To reflexognosists it is natural to link the major area of pressure around the metatarsophalangeal joints as depicted in body cavities on page 111. Pressure through this region is exacerbated by the pressure on locomotion. Reflexognosists can begin to relieve pressure in the feet through joint activation, stretching, working on the foot and leg, and developing a plan to strengthen the feet. In this way balance in the foot may take place. When this happens the energy is equally distributed in the foot and throughout the body. However, as soon as the client steps back into a pair of ill-fitting shoes, disharmony and imbalance result. This is usually accompanied by the experience of pain, pain which is often ignored.

High Heel Shoes

One of the distortions found in the foot that Dr. Wikler referred to was linked with congestion found in the chest plate of women brought about by wearing high heels. The way the foot locomotes in these shoes produces pressure at the metatarsal heads. The breast plate becomes congested and painful for many women. Direct anterior pressure constricts flow through the axilliary lymph. Secondly, the smaller toes receive no stimulation and are forced into an inactive position. The great toe takes all the pressure on the medial side. Normally, according to Wikler, the ten toes are like ten vital springs. In too many people the toes are permanently restricted and or dorsiflexed—and never touch the ground. The toes are so stiff they cannot be moved or spread. Tiredness, lethargy and fatigue, reduced peripheral vascular return, restricted muscle activity and congestive behavior in the thoracic cage occurs when this valuable resource of energy is lost.

Linking this to meridians, it is found most of the energy in the meridians will be reduced. Energy through the stomach meridian or the other meridians coming down through the feet will be reduced because the energy stops on the metatarsal heads, jarring through the foot. Biomechanically as the foot is hitting the ground there is too much pressure coming through the metatarsophalangeal joints. It is not equally distributed anywhere else. To reflexognosists the energy is totally locked causing physical and subtle energy congestion.

When high heels are worn, the angle on the foot applies pressure to the head of the metatarsophalangeal joints. From a podiatric viewpoint high-heeled shoes will propel the body onto the toes and the muscles in the front part of the body are stressed to compensate. This causes additional stress to the axilliary lymph and breast.

If the body is thrown anteriorly and excessive pressure is coming through the metatarsal heads, the reflexognosist, looking at the feet and super-imposing the anatomy over the feet, would say the tissue in the thoracic cavity is under pressure due to the body cavity stress. Wikler's studies have scientifically validated the concept of somatic replication of the forefoot to the thoracic cavity.

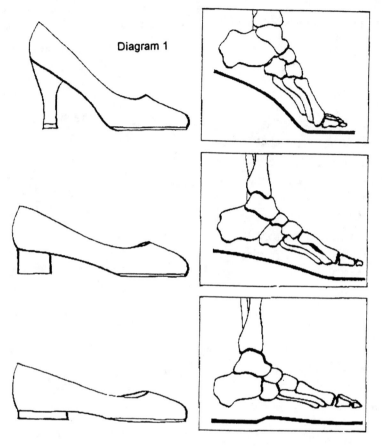

Diagram 1

Women's shoes are made for fashion and have very little to do with shape of the feet or how they work. The illustrations demonstrate the structural problems that develop from wearing certain heel heights. The pressure that is thrust on the forefoot in Diagram 1 causes the greatest concern. The results of extended wear are calluses and pinched nerves as well as foot and back pain. A study at Harvard Medical Schools in conjunction with The Spaulding Rehabilitation Hospital in Boston compared the force placed on joints when women walk barefoot and in 2 ½" heels. Dr. D. Casey Kerringan says the heels shift body weight forward increasing pressure on the knees by at least 23%. This may contribute to osteoarthritis of the knees, which is twice as common in women as men. The third shoe places the least possible stress on the foot. The low heel allows for a gentle tilt without placing stress on the anterior aspect of the foot and exposing the heads of the metatarsophalangeal joints. Wikler, however, warned against trying to change women who were accustomed to wearing high heels into flat shoes too quickly. Challenging the feet to normalcy too rapidly results in pain and the client could stop their program. The process to a correct shoe could take years.

As reflexognosists we must observe a person walking, look at their shoes and the condition of the feet as part of a session plan. The questions posed would be:

- Do the shoes they wear actually fit their feet?

- Are corns, calluses, bunions, and other deformities present?

If the shoes do not fit the feet, imagine what is happening. It must be remembered that no shoe, however perfect, will correct disabilities of the foot. Shoes that do not hinder the normal function of the joints and enhance muscle action simply provide the best environment in which the foot may work. Dr. Wikler contends in countries where people do not weaken and distort their feet by the shoes they wear, the population is largely immune to autoimmune or degenerative disorders.[3]

Because foot troubles are well on their way before the doctor is consulted and in the majority of cases are painless, the reflexognosist has a good opportunity to measure the client's foot for proper shoe size and provide exercises which may help support the very foundation of body structure and overall health. Remember—the primary function of the reflexognosist is to provide a stimulus to the body's innate intellect to heal from within and reduce the mechanical stress that results from poorly aligned feet.

The Wikler Foot Evaluation Protocol

Dr. Wikler found that if ten doctors examined one pair of feet they would make ten different determinations because there was no standard for foot evaluation. To combat this and for research purposes, Wikler designed the following nine assessments.[*] All of them taking less than five minutes. He suggested taking an initial assessment, keeping it on file and re-assessing periodically. The foot re-assessments will show foot improvement and progress.

1. Outer toe strength. Try to uncurl the client's toes as they provide resistance. All the muscles of your foot have to do with bending your toes. If you cannot bend your toes with strength, your foot muscles are weaker than good foot health would allow for. Toes should be as strong as your fingers. Can you uncurl the client's toes with your fingers? Can you bend their toes down?

2. Toe spreading. Using only the foot muscles, have the client spread their toes. Is there any or much space between them? Pointed shoes and rigid construction worn for years reduce the range of spread of the toes. Most shoe wearing people cannot spread or bend their toes fully. It is the breadth of spread which enables the entire body to keep in an easy balance.

3. Four outer toe deformity. Observe whether the toes are straight, curling, or abducting. Toe deformity and inefficiencies throw the mechanics of the entire body off balance and places the body under stress.

---

[*] Wikler's original foot evaluation chart, see page 134, has been modified by the authors.

4. Hallux valgus [bunion]. Is the head of the first metatarsal moved outward? The metatarsophalangeal joint of the great toe is an important lever to enable the body to propel itself forward. When the great toe is turned inward its leverage action is diminished. This leads to fatigue when standing or walking as the body requires greater physical energy to move forward.

5. Hip rotation. While the client is seated, grasp the client's feet and gently turn the toes to touch each other. Do not force this movement. Stop just short of discomfort. This tests the flexibility of the internal hip rotation.

6. Calf Contraction. The best way to test calf contraction is to have the client dorsiflex his foot as far as possible. A second way is to have the client, keeping the knees locked, bend from the waist and touch the toes. If one does not have supple calf muscles, walking will be stiff and not enjoyable.

Numbers 1-6 lend themselves to easy objectivity. Number 7 is a little more difficult to assess.

7. Foot pronation. [Refer to illustrations on page 109.] Ask the client to stand and check the foot posture. Is the long axis of the foot and leg on a straight sagittal line on both walking and standing? Or does the client lean on his inner arch with his weight resting on the inner arch perpetually?

8. Estimate muscle depth on the bottom of the foot. With your thumb on the dorsum, press your fingers into the plantar surface of the foot and feel how much muscle depth there is to the bone. A flat foot is usually a well muscled foot while a high arched foot usually has little muscle depth. Muscles are built by use and people who go barefooted often will have greater muscle depth.

9. Shoulder posture. Are the shoulders well back and squared with the head held level? Generally the person who goes barefooted will have good posture. For women, shoulder posture is especially important. When wearing high heels their posture is not balanced and as a result shoulders fall forward. This causes problems in the breast and axillary area.

A professional reflexognosist uses a protocol chart during the assessment phase of treatment to note what is observed.

Foot Exercises

It follows that the prevention and correction of foot disorders can be accomplished only when the tissues of the foot and the parts of the body vitally connected with the foot, are caused to function in the way that determines correct structure in the first place.

Specific foot exercises tend to prevent and overcome disorders in all parts of the body which apply especially to feet and legs. The natural forces of the body, whose business includes mending injured tissue, must be permitted to carry on its important work under the favorable influence of exercises that require the 'normal mode of activity' of joints and tissue.

FOOT PROTOCOL ASSESSMENT FORM
(Adapted from Dr. Simon J. Wikler's research protocol form)

Date _____ Social Security Number _____

Name _____ Age _____ Date of Birth _____

Address _____

_____ Phone _____

Size of shoe client wears _____ Size as measured _____

Client's evaluation of their feet _____

_____

Daily walking habits _____

Number of hours in socks or barefooted per day _____

Peripheral vascular return time _____

CRITERIA	SCORE		CRITERIA	SCORE		Code for Points
	R	L		R	L	Excellent - 4
1. Outer toes strength	____	____	6. Calf contraction	____	____	Fair - 3
2. Toe spreading	____	____	7. Foot pronation	____	____	Poor - 2
3. 4 outer toes deformity	____	____	8. Plantar muscle depth	____	____	Very poor - 1
4. Hallux valgus	____	____	9. Shoulder posture	____	____	Better feet 36-27
5. Movement of hips	____	____	TOTAL	____	____	Poor feet 26-19
						Very poor feet 9-18

Additional Notes:

The following exercises advocated by Wikler and others are designed to strengthen the foot. Exercises will vary with each client and be selected on weaknesses. Wikler felt between foot work and exercises, flexibility and range of movement would improve alone with circulation to all tissue in the foot.

Exercises complement and improve the effectiveness of hands-on work. Have the client do the exercises twice a day, and be re-checked several times a week initially, then taper off. The authors recommend for a weak or injured foot, *twice* the amount of exercise be performed as that given for the normal foot.

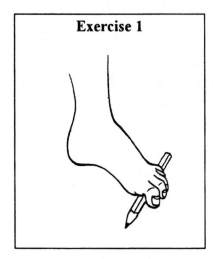

Exercise 1

Exercise rationale and instructions:
A person cannot walk well without proper toe strength. Muscles that move the toes are almost all the muscles of the entire foot. This exercise is designed to stretch the tendons on the dorsum of the foot. Sit in a relaxed position with the bare foot on the floor. Try to pick up a towel, marbles, or a pencil with the toes.

Movement:
The movement of the toes is a plantar flexion of the digits. Elevating the second phalanges on all digits.

Foot muscles activated:
Abductor hallucis, flexor digitorum brevis, quadratus plantae, lumbricals, flexor hallucis brevis, flexor digiti minimi brevis, dorsal interossei, plantar interossei, extensor hallucis brevis.

Leg muscles activated:
Flexor hallucis longus, tibialis posterior, extensor hallucis longus, tibialis anterior, extensor digitorum longus.

Physiological benefits:
- Increased stimulation of the circulatory and lymphatic systems
- Aid in relaxing the muscles in the lower leg and foot
- Increases the mobility of the joints in the metatarsals and phalanges

Reflexognosy benefits:
- Mobilization of the thoracic cavity and cervical spine area as somatically replicated on the foot
- Strengthens and increases flexibility in the toes for propulsion
- Increases the awareness and the usage of the toes
- Stretches the dorsal aspect of the foot

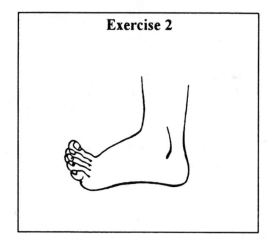

Exercise 2

Exercise rationale and instructions:
This exercise is designed to strengthen the toe muscles. Stand with the feet parallel and dorsiflex the toes up as far as possible. Repeat several times.

Movement:
This is a dorsiflexion of the toes at the metatarsophalangeal joints.

Foot muscles activated:
Abductor hallucis, flexor digitorum brevis, abductor digiti minimi, lumbricals, dorsal interossei, plantar interossei, extensor digitorum brevis, extensor hallucis brevis.

Leg muscles activated:
Extensor hallucis longus, peroneus tertius, extensor digitorum longus.

Physiological benefits:
- Stimulation of circulatory and lymphatic systems
- Strengthening of the dorsal aspect of the foot
- Strengthening of the anterior compartment of the leg

Reflexognosy benefits:
- Increased awareness of the toes
- Stimulation to the cranial cavity

Alternate Toe Exercises:

2A. Sit with the toes dorsiflexed. Curl the toes under and squeeze them together for 5 seconds using only the muscles in the foot. Rest and repeat. This exercise can be modified by grabbing the curled toes with the fingers and trying to uncurl the clenched toes while the toes resist.

2B. While sitting, place a thick rubber band around all the toes of one foot. Spread the toes apart as far as possible and hold for five seconds. Switch feet and repeat.

2C. Walk on the toes without letting the heels touch the ground. This strengthens not only the toes but the shins and stretches the calf muscles.

2D. Walk on the heels holding the toes high off the ground. This strengthens the shins and stretches the calf muscles.

2E. Sit with the feet flat on the floor. Raise the heel of one foot slowly; hold for 5 seconds. Rest and repeat.

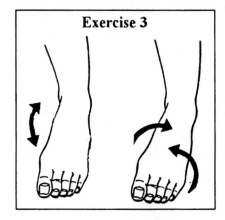

Exercise 3

Exercise rationale and instructions:
This exercise is designed to relieve stiffness of the ankle joint. Sit is a chair with one leg crossed over the other. Bend the foot down and then up. Rotate the foot in one direction and then in the other. Repeat 10-15 times.

Movement:
The movement is a plantar flexion and dorsiflexion of the ankle joint coupled with the inverting and everting of the same joint.

Foot muscles activated:
Flexor digitorum brevis, abductor digiti minimi, quadratus plantae, lumbricals.

Leg muscles activated:
Flexor hallucis longus, tibialis posterior, plantaris, flexor digitorum longus, gastrocnemius, soleus, peroneus longus, peroneus brevis, extensor hallucis longus, peroneus tertius, tibialis anterior, extensor digitorum longus.

Physiological benefits:
- Stimulation of the circulatory and lymphatic systems
- Increased flexibility in the muscular and skeletal systems.

Reflexognosy benefits:
- Stretching of the connective tissue
- Relaxation of the plantar fascia
- Increased strength and locomotion skills.

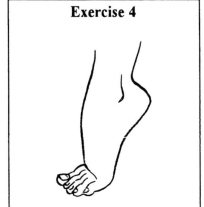

Exercise 4

Exercise rationale and instructions:
This exercise is to relieve rigidity in the ankle and the longitudinal arch. Alternately stand flat on your feet and raise to your toes. Do this several times.

Movement:
In this position the ankle joint is again being plantar flexed and inverted.

Foot muscles activated:
Abductor hallucis, flexor digitorum brevis, abductor digiti minimi, lumbricals, flexor digiti minim brevis, dorsal interossei, plantar interossei, extensor digitorum brevis, extensor hallucis brevis.

Leg muscles activated:
Flexor hallucis longus, tibialis posterior, plantaris, flexor digitorum longus, gastrocnemius, soleus, peroneus longus, peroneus brevis, extensor hallucis longus, peroneus tertius, tibialis anterior, extensor digitorum longus.

Physiological benefits:
- Stimulation of the circulatory and lymphatic systems
- Increased flexibility and relaxation of the musculature of the leg and foot.

Reflexognosy benefits:
- Stimulation of the thoracic and cranial cavities
- Increased flexibility in the thoracic and cervical spinal reflex areas
- Increased strength of the longitudinal and transverse arches in the foot.

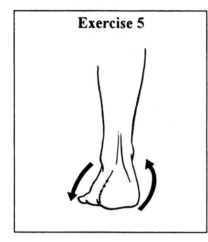

Exercise 5

Exercise rationale and instructions:
This exercise is designed to relieve strain on the two inner longitudinal arches. Roll the feet outwards fifteen or twenty times so that the weight rests on the outer border of the feet.

Movement:
Inversion of the foot and ankle.

Foot muscles activated:
Abductor hallucis, dorsal interossei, plantar interossei, extensor digitorum brevis.

Leg muscles activated:
Flexor hallucis longus, flexor digitorum longus, gastrocnemius, soleus, peroneus longus, peroneus brevis, tibialis anterior, extensor digitorum longus.

Physiological benefits:
- Stimulation of the lymphatic and circulatory systems
- Increased ankle joint stability and strength
- Decrease of flat feet—supination will increase arch depth
- Increase of balance

Reflexognosy benefits:
- Help relax plantar fascia and arches
- Stimulates all body cavities

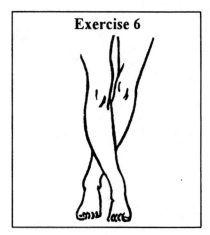

Exercise 6

Exercise rationale and instructions:
This exercise is designed to utilize every muscle used in balance. Stand stiff-kneed with the legs crossed like scissors. The feet are parallel and slightly apart so that the weight of the body is distributed evenly on both feet. Hold the position for a minute or two. Rest and then repeat several times.

Movement:
Inversion of the feet.

Foot muscles activated:
Abductor hallucis, flexor digitorum brevis, abductor digiti minimi, quadratus plantae, lumbricals, dorsal interossei, plantar interossei, extensor digitorum brevis, extensor hallucis brevis.

Leg muscles activated:
Flexor hallucis longus, tibialis posterior, flexor digitorum longus, gastrocnemius, soleus, extensor hallucis longus, peroneus tertius, tibialis anterior, extensor digitorum longus.

Physiological benefits:
- Assists in reversing pelvic or femoral rotation
- Stimulation to the circulatory, lymphatic, muscular, skeletal, and nervous systems

Reflexognosy benefits:
- Assists those who heavily pronate to increase supination
- Increases support and stability of the body
- Stretches plantar fascia and longitudinal arches

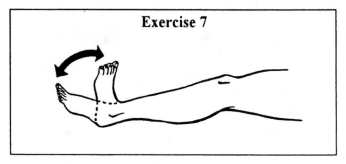

Exercise 7

Exercise rationale and instructions:
This exercise is designed to strengthen the muscles of the calf and the heel. Sit on the floor with the legs straight ahead and dorsiflex the feet as far as possible

Movement:
The movement is a dorsiflexion of the ankles and toes.

Foot muscles activated:
Flexor digitorum brevis, lumbricals, flexor hallucis brevis, flexor digiti minimi brevis, dorsal interossei, plantar interossei, extensor digitorum brevis, extensor hallucis brevis.

Leg muscles activated:
Flexor hallucis longus, tibialis posterior, plantaris, flexor digitorum longus, gastrocnemius, soleus, peroneus longus, peroneus brevis, extensor hallucis longus, tibialis anterior, extensor digitorum longus.

Physiological benefits:
• Stretching of the musculature
• Stimulation of the circulatory and lymphatic systems.

Reflexognosy benefits:
• Strengthens the muscles in the anterior compartment
• Assists in prevention of shin splints

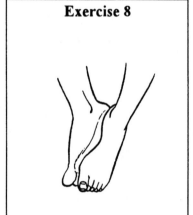
Exercise 8

Exercise rationale and instructions:
This exercise is designed to strengthen the arch and tone the calf. Sit with the legs straight ahead. Turn the soles of the feet together. If only the heels and medial sides of the great toe touch, modify the exercise by bending the knees.

Movement:
Inversion and plantar flexion.

Foot muscles activated:
flexor digitorum brevis, quadratus plantae, lumbricals, flexor hallucis brevis, dorsal interossei, plantar interossei, extensor digitorum brevis, extensor hallucis brevis.

Leg muscles activated:
Flexor hallucis longus, tibialis posterior, plantaris, flexor digitorum longus, peroneus longus, peroneus brevis, extensor hallucis longus, tibialis anterior, extensor digitorum longus.

Physiological benefits:
• Strengthens musculature of the pelvic area, leg and foot
• Increases ankle flexibility

Reflexognosy benefits:
• With legs straight and heels and great toes touching, stimulation in the lumbar, sacral, and cervical spine reflexes

- With both feet together and knees slightly bent, all four cavities will be stimulated.

Alternative Exercises:

8A. Walk on the lateral edges of the feet while concentrating on holding the ankles steady. This exercise develops the calves and stretches the tendons running around the lateral malleolus.

8B. Walk on the medial edges of the feet, trying to keep the lateral edge off the ground. This strengthens shins and the small ankle stabilizing leg muscles.

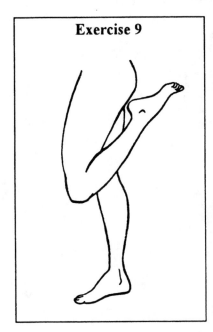

Exercise 9

Exercise rationale and instructions:
This exercise is designed to stretch the thigh muscles. Face a wall. Lean against a wall with your weight on your arms. Kick yourself in the buttock.

Movement:
This is a knee-flexion movement

Foot muscles activated:
Flexor digitorum brevis, quadratus plantae, extensor digitorum brevis.

Leg muscles activated:
Flexor digitorum longus, gastrocnemius, soleus, peroneus longus, peroneus brevis, extensor digitorum longus.

Physiological Benefits:
- Increase of muscle tone
- Balances excessive pronation by strengthening supination
- Increased stimulation to circulatory and lymphatic systems

Reflexognosy benefits:
- All compartments of the extrinsic muscles are involved in balancing the foot placed on the ground
- The intrinsic muscles act as accessories to stabilize and balance the body
- All body cavities in contact with the floor are stimulated.

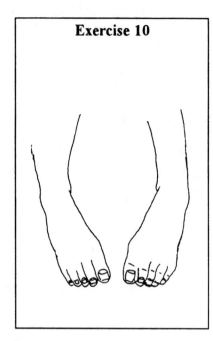

Exercise 10

Exercise rationale and instructions:
This exercise is designed to limber up the hips and ankles. Walk with the feet turned in as far as possible (pigeon-toed). This may be alternated by walking with the feet turned out as far as possible (duck waddle).

Movement:
This is a hip rotation movement

Foot muscles activated:
All muscles are activated when performed strongly.

Leg muscles activated:
All compartments are involved when performed strongly.

Physiological benefits:
- Assists in reversing pelvic or femoral rotation
- Stimulation to the circulatory, lymphatic, muscular, skeletal and nervous systems

Reflexognosy benefits:
- Assists those who heavily pronate to increase supination or the reverse.
- Increases support and stability of the body
- Stretches plantar fascia and longitudinal arches

These ten exercises will strengthen and stretch all of the muscles of the feet and legs, and will help prevent ankle sprains, Achilles tendon problems, shin soreness and plantar fasciitis. The walking exercises should be begun slowly walking 10 yards in each of the four positions. Walk 40 yards normally, and then repeat the exercises for another 40 yards. As the client becomes stronger the exercises can be repeated three and four times. For the seated exercises repeat each exercise ten times. The client should never push with any of these exercises but stop at the point undue strain is felt.

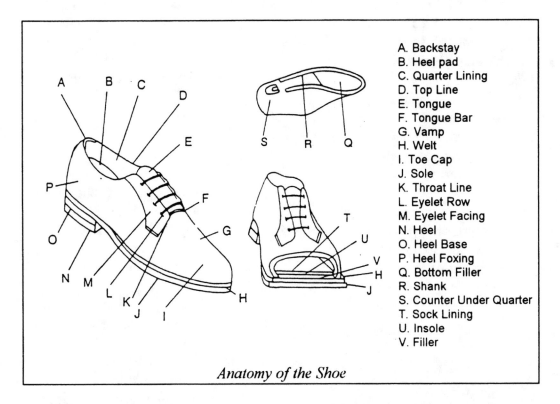

A. Backstay
B. Heel pad
C. Quarter Lining
D. Top Line
E. Tongue
F. Tongue Bar
G. Vamp
H. Welt
I. Toe Cap
J. Sole
K. Throat Line
L. Eyelet Row
M. Eyelet Facing
N. Heel
O. Heel Base
P. Heel Foxing
Q. Bottom Filler
R. Shank
S. Counter Under Quarter
T. Sock Lining
U. Insole
V. Filler

Anatomy of the Shoe

The Perfect Shoe

Properly fitting footwear is an important aspect to good foot health. The application of reflexognosy will help general health, but when the client puts his or her foot back into an ill-fitting pair of shoes, the work just completed can easily be undone with the first few steps he or she takes. Reflexognosists can educate their clients about the importance of their shoes and how to obtain the best fit possible.

The simple reason shoes distort the feet is because they are not the same shape as the feet. Dr. Wikler told those who studied with him not to waste time trying to find the perfect shoe. None exist. The best thing to do during the work day was wear whatever was appropriate for their occupation that fitted properly, but around the house compensate for this by wearing slipper socks or going barefooted. He found the simple old-fashioned canvas tennis shoe, not the jogging shoe, to be the best because of its flexibility. Leading researcher, Steven Robbins, M.D., of Montreal General Hospital concurs. He explains that with a "thick, cushiony sole, it's more difficult to judge the angle of your foot in relation to the ground. Your foot could be on a sharp tilt, for example, but the supersized sole makes it feel as though your foot is planted flatly on the surface you're walking on. Thus, you might think your whole foot has hit the ground when in fact only the foot's edge has touched down. That misperception can seriously impede balance and lead to falls."[1] This also forces the ankle tendons to contract more to maintain balance, which in turn, reduces the ankle's ability to sense your foot position. The article also suggests the lack of sensitivity is especially relevant for older people.

While some experts feel the foot should be kept in rigid alignment, Wikler disagreed. He felt restricted foot movement did not allow for the natural exercise of the foot. Once again, Robbins agrees, but takes things a step further. "People in hard-soled shoes, such as racing sneakers with thin bottoms, run or walk with more of a bend in the knee and also more of a bend at the hip. That causes them to sink a little closer to the ground, which gives much more shock absorption value than what any spongy material in the sole would provide."[3]

Orthotics

Wikler disapproved of orthotics because they limited movement. However, with the advances in orthotics today which now allow the foot to move naturally, Wikler may be of a different opinion. Correct fitting of orthoses is important. They should be checked and adjusted frequently because the feet will change between the work the practitioner and client do.

Shoe Sizing

There are no two shoe styles alike in terms of size. Different shoes in identical sizes and widths will measure and fit differently. The reasons for this inconsistency are many:

1. Style affects size

2. Heel height affects size

3. Materials can affect size

4. Patterns or the 'cut' will affect size

5. Lasts affect size

6. Construction affects size

7. Shoe manufacturers influence size by making up their own sizing

Consequently it is always best to try on shoes before purchasing them, paying close attention to fit rather than size.

Lasts

The last of the shoe is the wooden or metal form on which the shoe is shaped. It should conform to the shape of the foot. If not, the foot and the shoe will not function properly. This can cause irritation to the foot and improper wear to the shoe. The last varies according to country of origin. Asian lasts are wider than Italian and French lasts, which are narrower than German ones. American and German lasts are about equal and English lasts are larger.

The feet below are the same length from the heel to the toe, however each would require a different shoe size. The measurement from ball to heel is not the same. The ball of the shoe is the widest part of the shoe, and the ball of the foot is the widest part of the foot. These two areas should coincide.

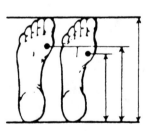

Same length of foot with different heel to ball measurement which requires different size of shoes.

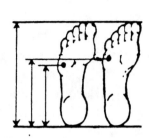

Same length of foot with different heel to 5ᵗʰ metatarsal measurement which requires different size of shoes.

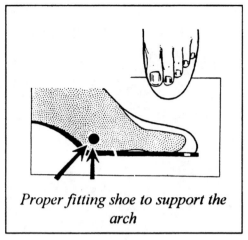

Proper fitting shoe to support the arch

In the illustration above, the feet are once again the same length from heel to toe and also from heel to the ball of the foot, however, the measurements on the lateral side of the foot at the head of the 5th metatarsal are different. In order for a shoe to fit properly, these three points on the foot—the heads of the first and fifth metatarsals and the longitudinal arch—must all coincide.

If the shoe does not fit properly it will not support the foot in the longitudinal arch. As the foot moves forward, this puts pressure on the metatarsal heads and the tips of the toes while it pinches the toes in the edge of the narrow toe box. The proper fit on the right supports the longitudinal arch, however a wider toe box would be better.

Correctly Fitting Shoes

While a proper fit in shoes is critical, the medical profession, the average shoe sales person, and consumers do not know what constitutes a proper fit. Measuring your client's feet for shoe size is a valuable service you can provide for them. Remember: fit the shoe to the foot; do not force the foot to conform to the shoe!

The correctly fitting shoe will allow room for the foot to move so that the intrinsic anatomy of the foot is able to perform the vital function of movement. Circulation will improve and the nervous system will respond to the stimulus of locomotion improving overall health.

The place to fit a shoe is not at the end of the toes, but across the ball of the foot. To determine the proper size of a shoe one can use a Brannock Measuring device which can conveniently measure the arch length, the width at the head of the first metatarsal, and the overall length. A simple ruler can measure length, or a piece of paper can also be used to check length and width. You or your client can draw the shape of the foot on a piece of paper. Then place the shoe over the outline.

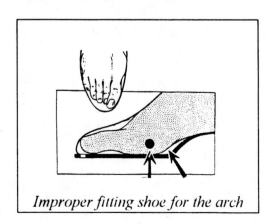

Improper fitting shoe for the arch

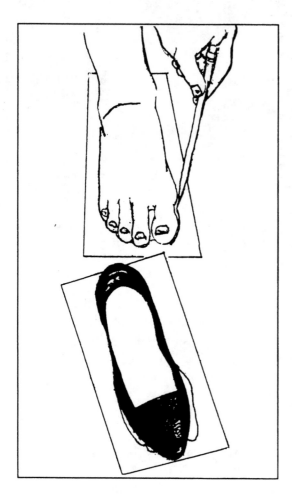

If the ball of the foot, or any other area, overhangs the sides of the shoe, the foot is being squeezed and either a wider or longer shoe is called for.

Looking at the wear pattern on the sole can also indicate where the gait is heaviest or where the foot is not touching the ground, and whether there is excessive pronation or supination.

Shoes For Everyday Wear

Generally, for everyday wear, for both men and women lace-ups are best as they can be longer and wider, giving the foot adequate room, maintaining foot comfort throughout the day, while the shoe stays on the foot.

When you choose shoes with many eyelets you can customize the fit. It is simply a matter of how they are laced. For instance with a high arch, lace the shoes straight across the tongue without a crisscross pattern. If the second toe is longer than the great toe, or hammertoes or corns are present, the joints in the effected toes may bend upward and get sore if your shoes are laced too tight. In this case, to relieve pressure in the toe box, lace from the inside front eyelet to the opposite last eyelet.

Shopping for a Custom Fit

1. Have the feet measured *every* time a pair of shoes is purchased. Feet grow with age. In addition, about 80% of all pregnant women's feet grow one half shoe size. A woman with several children may have grown a full size or more due to the hormones that relax the pelvis in preparation for birth. They also can act to relax and elongate the feet. Despite growth, heel size generally stays the same, but the front of the foot becomes wider and longer. The result is that many women wear shoes that fit at the heel but are too narrow or short in the front. A recent study of 255 women revealed that to get a snugger fit in the heel, 73% wore athletic shoes that were too tight in the forefoot. Men also wear shoes too small—usually by two sizes.

2. **Do not let the salesperson 'customize the fit'** by putting pads in the shoes. When doing so the pair truly does not fit. Be sure the inner seams do not rub against the foot. The worst advice given is that shoes will stretch after they have been worn for awhile.

Shoes should fit properly in the store!

3. Shop for shoes at the end of the day, when feet are largest. The volume of feet can increase by 5-10% during a workout or during the course of the day.

Special Advice for the Sports Enthusiast

Concordia University in Montreal reports that expensive running shoes which promise extra cushioning and 'pronation correction' may cause more injuries than moderately priced shoes. Shoes that absorb too much impact mask the sensation of the feet hitting the ground and keep the person from reacting to subtle pain signals that tell the sports enthusiast when to modify techniques to prevent injuries.

Replace athletic shoes by mileage or number of hours logged rather than by signs of wear and tear. Usually the cushion of the inner midsole, which cannot be seen is the first to wear out. It is recommended to replace running shoes every 500 miles; walking shoes every 500-700 miles and aerobics shoes or cross-trainers after 100 hours of wear.

Enthusiasts should simulate their sport in the store. For instance in tennis shoes lung from side to side, or jog in place if a runner.

Socks

Socks were also another area of concern for Wikler. Oftentimes socks and stockings are tight, compressing the feet all day long. He did not like pantyhose because of their restrictive qualities. Wikler also did not appreciate the sizes of stockings today and felt there should be more sizes to choose from so that stockings could be roomy, but not too spacious. Many people wear socks that have shrunk from too many washings, which could cause toes to curl under and could accelerate an already existing problem like hammertoes. Super stretchy hosiery can have the same effect; be sure to stretch hose as you put them on to give toes needed room. Select socks of natural fibers such as cotton or wool. When trying on shoes, whatever the sport or activity, always wear the appropriate socks that will be worn with the shoes to get the best fit.

Shoe Material

Leather is still the best upper material, with canvas a close second. A closed vinyl shoe is the worst. Feet must be allowed to breathe, and synthetic materials, such as vinyl, prevent that. If you wear vinyl or nylon, choose a mesh design that will provide some ventilation.

Writes Wikler (1990) in *A Guide to Foot Assessment for Reflexologists*, "The work you are doing as a reflexologist is the most important work being done for a person's health. ...What is most attractive to me about your profession is that you practice hands-on techniques with the feet. Second, that you spend 30 to 45 minutes of continuous tissue manipulations of the feet in your usual treatment. Third, a basic tenet of your profession is that affectations of the feet are closely allied to total health."

"It is the most natural thing

that healing arts should work with you. But only the will of the members of your profession can organize the additional skills needed to make reflexologists part of the healing arts fraternity. This will ultimately include schools with increased curriculums and licensure by state governments,"[4] he concluded.

A central feature of training in reflexognosy focuses on the important role footwear plays in the health of the feet, and is a vital consideration when pain is found within the foot. Reflexognosists have followed Wikler's lead in visually assessing the foot, educating clients on what constitutes a good shoe, and providing exercises which strengthen the foot and its function. They have taken the advice of Wikler and will continue to do so as the profession develops. In addition, the curriculum of Reflexognosy is constantly being upgraded as new information and skills relevant to the feet are researched.

---

[1] Wikler, Simon. *A Guide to Foot Assessment for Reflexologists*, Sacramento CA, 1990, pg. 17.
[2] Robbins, Steven. An article in *Health & Nutrition Letter* from Tufts University. April 1997, vol. 15, No. 2
[3] Ibid.
[4] Wikler, Simon, pg. 1.

Chapter 12

Physiological Response to Reflexognosy

Nothing is contrary to the laws of nature, only to what we understand about the laws of nature.

—St. Thomas Aquinas

While the technological approach of conventional medicine, which focuses on control of an offending part of the body is important, it must be balanced with tactile therapies which have practitioners trained to focus on the entire person. The tactile therapist on the other hand, must balance their hands-on skills with an understanding of how their therapy works.

In order to answer the question of what happens physiologically during a reflexognosy session we must start at the very beginning with the process of communication. Without the communication pathway there can be no response. For reflexognosy to work on a physical level there must be a way for the body, through the feet, to detect a stimulus. When looking at the physical structure of the foot the first layer seen is the skin. The

thickness of the layer is far less on the upper or dorsal aspect of the foot than on the plantar or bottom of the foot. The thicker layers are for additional protection. In the feet and hands there are many sensory receptors. There are many classifications of receptors, but proprioceptors and exteroceptors will be mentioned here.

A proprioceptor is any of the sensory nerves that give information concerning movements and position of the body; they occur chiefly in muscles, tendons and the labyrinth [inner ear]. This definition of proprioceptors explains how the use of biomechanical principles has an influence on the effectiveness of reflexognosy. The way we transfer our weight from one part of our foot to the other stimulates these receptors in the muscles and other tissue in our feet.

Exteroceptors, which are located near the surface of the body in the skin, transmit impulses of touch, pressure and pain; they are also important. In reflexognosy, touch, pressure and pain or sensitivity, is the body's way of communicating with the distal parts of the body.

The Peripheral Nervous System consists of nerves and ganglion outside the brain and spinal cord. It links the Central Nervous System with the body's receptors—sensory cells and sense organs—and all parts of the body such as muscles and glands that respond to nerve impulse instruction from the Central Nervous System.

The stimulus applied by the reflexognosist is picked up by the various sensory nerves in the feet and transferred to the spinal cord and brain for processing. In the spinal cord the impulse transfers via the interneurons to the preganglionic nerves of the autonomic nervous system, from here to the viscera, or organs, blood vessels, and glandular tissue. This *process* is called a visceral autonomic reflex—a response to a stimulus. The process has been charted according to the connection of the vertebrae to nerves of the sympathetic and parasympathetic system. Included in the chart [see page 145] are some conditions which are produced when interference with the nerves is created by pressure.

The same impulse can travel through the brain stem and on to the hypothalamus. The hypothalamus provides us with a link between the nervous and hormonal systems. The brain stem also contains the medulla oblongata that is an integral part of the autonomic

nervous system. Through the pathway of the body's interrelationship, the entire structure responds to the stimulation created by the reflexognosist.

Rossi and Cheek (1994) offer an in-depth answer to the question: Why do we achieve such profound results when working on the feet and legs?

"The cortical-limbic-hypothalamic system is thus the major locus for integrating the sensory-perceptual stimuli selected for attention with the regulation of the autonomic, endocrine, and immune systems by the hypothalamic-pituitary system. That is, signals received by the opiate receptors at the limbic-hypothalamic level modulate the major channel of mind-body information transduction between the sensory-perceptual and memory systems with the autonomic, endocrine, and immune systems that are of essence in homeostasis and psychosomatic problems. Since the entire cortical-limbic-hypothalamic system is in a constant state of psychobiological flux, the state of dependent memory and learning systems they encode are in similar flux. The stability of memory and learning that we depend upon for daily living is actually a precarious illusion that is dependent upon the degree to which psychobiological homeostasis is maintained in the cortical-limbic-hypothalamic-pituitary system."[1]

Due to the fact reflexognoists affect these areas with stimulus to the feet is, in part, an answer to our basic question. The authors of the above texts add further information about the peri-

150

CHART OF EFFECTS OF SPINAL MISALIGNMENTS

"The nervous system controls and coordinates all organs and structures of the human body." (*Gray's Anatomy*, 29th Ed., page 4). Misalignments of spinal vertebrae and discs may cause irritation to the nervous system and affect the structures, organs, and functions which may result in the conditions shown below.

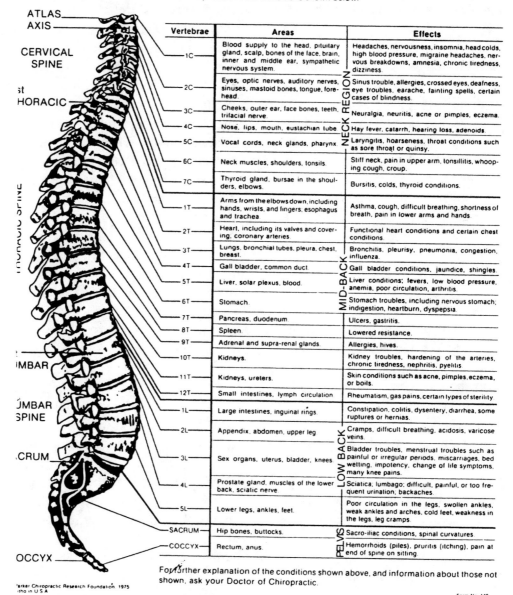

Vertebrae	Areas	Effects
1C	Blood supply to the head, pituitary gland, scalp, bones of the face, brain, inner and middle ear, sympathetic nervous system.	Headaches, nervousness, insomnia, head colds, high blood pressure, migraine headaches, nervous breakdowns, amnesia, chronic tiredness, dizziness.
2C	Eyes, optic nerves, auditory nerves, sinuses, mastoid bones, tongue, forehead.	Sinus trouble, allergies, crossed eyes, deafness, eye troubles, earache, fainting spells, certain cases of blindness.
3C	Cheeks, outer ear, face bones, teeth, trifacial nerve.	Neuralgia, neuritis, acne or pimples, eczema.
4C	Nose, lips, mouth, eustachian tube.	Hay fever, catarrh, hearing loss, adenoids.
5C	Vocal cords, neck glands, pharynx.	Laryngitis, hoarseness, throat conditions such as sore throat or quinsy.
6C	Neck muscles, shoulders, tonsils.	Stiff neck, pain in upper arm, tonsillitis, whooping cough, croup.
7C	Thyroid gland, bursae in the shoulders, elbows.	Bursitis, colds, thyroid conditions.
1T	Arms from the elbows down, including hands, wrists, and fingers, esophagus and trachea.	Asthma, cough, difficult breathing, shortness of breath, pain in lower arms and hands.
2T	Heart, including its valves and covering, coronary arteries.	Functional heart conditions and certain chest conditions.
3T	Lungs, bronchial tubes, pleura, chest, breast.	Bronchitis, pleurisy, pneumonia, congestion, influenza.
4T	Gall bladder, common duct.	Gall bladder conditions, jaundice, shingles.
5T	Liver, solar plexus, blood.	Liver conditions, fevers, low blood pressure, anemia, poor circulation, arthritis.
6T	Stomach.	Stomach troubles, including nervous stomach, indigestion, heartburn, dyspepsia.
7T	Pancreas, duodenum.	Ulcers, gastritis.
8T	Spleen.	Lowered resistance.
9T	Adrenal and supra-renal glands.	Allergies, hives.
10T	Kidneys.	Kidney troubles, hardening of the arteries, chronic tiredness, nephritis, pyelitis.
11T	Kidneys, ureters.	Skin conditions such as acne, pimples, eczema, or boils.
12T	Small intestines, lymph circulation.	Rheumatism, gas pains, certain types of sterility.
1L	Large intestines, inguinal rings.	Constipation, colitis, dysentery, diarrhea, some ruptures or hernias.
2L	Appendix, abdomen, upper leg.	Cramps, difficult breathing, acidosis, varicose veins.
3L	Sex organs, uterus, bladder, knees.	Bladder troubles, menstrual troubles such as painful or irregular periods, miscarriages, bed wetting, impotency, change of life symptoms, many knee pains.
4L	Prostate gland, muscles of the lower back, sciatic nerve.	Sciatica, lumbago; difficult, painful, or too frequent urination, backaches.
5L	Lower legs, ankles, feet.	Poor circulation in the legs, swollen ankles, weak ankles and arches, cold feet, weakness in the legs, leg cramps.
SACRUM	Hip bones, buttocks.	Sacro-iliac conditions, spinal curvatures.
COCCYX	Rectum, anus.	Hemorrhoids (piles), pruritis (itching), pain at end of spine on sitting.

For further explanation of the conditions shown above, and information about those not shown, ask your Doctor of Chiropractic.

Parker Chiropractic Research Foundation, 1975
Litho in U.S.A.

Form No. 149

Chart 4

aqueductal gray region of the brain stem which provides some understanding. "This brain stem area is another well known locus where opiate analgesia is mediated. (Pert & Yaksh. 1974). Pert (1980) has noted that it is in direct point-to-point synaptic communication with the 'frontal cortex and is thus thought to mediate the well-documented effect of expectation and conscious control on pain perception.'"

This is directly aligned to reflexognosists. We have an influence on the brain stem and this quote offers answers, in part, to questions posed pertaining to the mechanism by which results are achieved.

Pain Relief

Pain relieving chemicals such as endorphins have been located in the pituitary. Their relevance to reflexognosy is that they stop the impulses in the pain pathway providing an analgesic effect. Endorphins are said to have an anti-depressant effect also. When a reflexognosist applies pressure to the feet, the endorphin level is triggered as the nervous system interprets this stimulus, as well as setting up communication with the periaqueductal gray region of the brain stem as discussed above.

Enkephalins are also natural pain killers associated with pain pathways. They too will be stimulated when the pain stimulus is processed. Endorphins are said to be 200 times more powerful than morphine and are being researched for possible pain control. Neuropeptides are being discovered con-

stantly. No doubt there will be many more natural pain relieving substances coming to light in the future.

Following a session, the client may feel sedated, euphoric or experience mood swings. It is theorized that endorphins, as natural mood enhancers, play a part in this response. Also the neurotransmitter, Gamma aminobutyric acid, or GABA, which is located in the hypothalmus as well as the thalmus has been found to be the body's natural valium. When the action of GABA has been enhanced, the response is mood elevation, which acts as an anti-depressant, calming the person. Reflexognosy may increase the GABA levels in the body and this is one aspect that is attributed to the feeling of profound relaxation during and following a session generally.

Pain Tolerance

Practitioners have a dual physiological and ethical responsibility not to exceed the client's pain threshold. When the reflexognosist comes in contact with the elaborate nerve pathways in the feet, complex messages have gone to the brain and back again. If the pressing produces pain it is a different sensation coming through the sensory nervous system. Physiologically a high percentage of healing is immediately negated when the practitioner exceeds the client's pain threshold. The diaphragm/solar plexus tightens. The autonomic nerve ganglia is suppressed by the activation of the musculature that is stressed due to the pain sensation recorded through the spine. This slows the sensory pathways, circulation and lymphatic supply and endorphin production may be reduced. This action then becomes counter productive.

Touch

Finally, the sensation of touch effects the brain in a unique way. The region of the brain where sensations of temperature, pain, and touch are perceived is the sensory cortex of the parietal lobe. There is a crossover in the pathways of sensation from the body before the brain is reached. The sensory nerves cross either in the spinal cord or in the brain stem so that sensations for the left side of the body reach the sensory cortex of the right cerebral hemisphere and those from the right side of the body are registered in the left cortex. The strip of sensory cortex in one hemisphere is duplicated in the other hemisphere. Each region of the body sends signals that reach a fairly well-defined area of the sensory cortex.

While this may indicate a crossover of responses to a degree, the fact that the brain and the sensory receptors adapt to the sensation of pressure very quickly may account for any limited crossover effect the practitioner may observe. It would appear that another avenue of stimulation is used by the body when dealing with reflexognosy.

Words like neurotransmitter, proprioceptors, sensory cortex, and autonomic pathways are areas that will provide answers for the reflexognosist. The affects of Reflexognosy, in part, can be explained from the medical model with a firm understanding of anatomy and physiology. It should be noted that this is but one model and the reflexognosist will search out many models to explain the wholistic outcomes that are achieved during and following sessions. The pure physiological responses to the application of reflexognosy can be clearly defined but investigation must continue as only some of the answers are currently available.

Systems of the Body

Reflexognosy affects the cardiovascular system with no additional strain on the heart. Reflexognosy stimulates the lymphatic system via the feet which brings about a physiological change to the entire immune system. The lymphatic system is not reliant on the pumping from the heart, but on activity. With reflexognosy the feet are encouraged to mimic activity and will affect the body accordingly. The anatomy housed in the feet is stimulated: the fascia, ligaments, muscles, tendons, blood vessels, and the lymphatic vessels. Congestion in lymph areas, such as the axilla in the arm pits and the groin region, may be cleared through enhanced functioning. By working the lymphatics in one part of the body, flow is promoted. In clearing congestion in the lymphatic system the circulatory and lymphatic systems work in harmony with each other.

Reflexognosy deals with three different branches of the nervous systems: the autonomic, central, and sensory nervous systems. The influence from the feet stimulates messages back to the brain, transferring through the spinal column, and out through the autonomic nerve ganglia. This is an integral aspect of reflexognosy.

To move your body is a function of the central nervous system. For organs to operate is the function of the autonomic nervous system, but all innervation radiates from the spine. Stimulation can be manifested in the feet, through the rest of the body to the brain. No part of the body works in isolation. Any influence around the feet is going to affect the entire nervous system. Structure and function work in tandem to produce balance and harmony for the healing process to begin.

The autonomic nerve ganglia works via the spinal column, but sits outside of it, and is a major influence on the nerve supply to the body. If someone had a problem with T-5, poor circulation and liver conditions/congestion could be present. Biomechanical deviations from normalcy in the feet will adversely affect the spinal column and will affect the autonomic nerve ganglia and will, by extension, have a role to play in organ dysfunction.

Chiropractors base their work on this link. A study was conducted by Henry Winsor, M.D. (1921) with autopsies, which support the claim that there is a relationship between visceral disease and vertebral deformities of the same sympathetic segments. This research was of 50 cadavers examined and found to have diseases in 139 organs. All curves and deformities of the spine were noted. It was found there was a curve of the vertebrae belonging to the same sympathetic segments as the dis-

eased organs 128 times! Of the other 11 it was found that the vertebrae in curve belonged to an adjacent segment to that which should supply the diseased organs with sympathetic filament. This makes sense when one remembers that an organ may receive sympathetic filaments from several spinal segments. In essence, the researchers found in *100%* of the cases the vertebra that was out of alignment was tied to the organ whose dysfunction was the cause of death.[2] Eunice Ingham was well aware of this connection when she wrote, "A misplaced vertebra, in any part of the spine, will be sure to cut off the normal circulation and interfere with the contracting and relaxing of the part which is depending upon this particular nerve for its blood supply."[3] The reflexognosist will focus on this link, observing structural deviations from normalcy within the feet and assess pressure within the spinal area and its affects on the related organ.

Dermatomes

Working with the medical model, the other area reflexognosy has a major influence on, are the dermatomes of the body. Dermatomes are segmental skin areas innervated by various spinal cord segments. These are different than those innervated by the autonomic nerve ganglia. Through dermatomes there is an influence to the external parts of our body on the skin. It has been found a light stretching brings about changes in the internal functioning of the body. Why? Because, light stretching touch has an influence on derma-

154

tomal function which has an influence on the organs of the body. We can have an influence on the dermatomal function merely by touch.

This rationale is based on the medical model. This is not to say that the entire model is correct in all areas but reflexognosists are

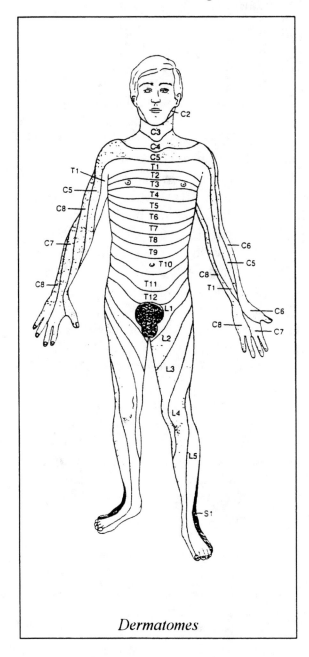

Dermatomes

aware of the areas that have credibility and the above are in this domain. From a strictly physiological perspective they help in under-

standing some of the mechanisms by which reflexognosy works.

Emotional Level

As reflexognosists we touch people on many levels—physically, emotionally, mentally and spiritually, through our hands and communication skills. Feelings are part of the mind/body connection. In the body, feelings include the physical sensation of touch and incorporate the emotions. With the application of touch and pressure to the feet messages are physically sent to the brain through the nervous system and elicit a physical response. Other messages are also communicated to the client silently through our hands, tactile skills, our voice, our attitude towards life, our intentions, etc. Touch can be curative when we touch someone with healing and love in mind. Through this multi-level reaction to touch the client often has an opportunity to experience a sense of security, trust and well-being from which new coping skills may develop. The client may learn new ways of approaching his/her world simply by being touched. Therefore, the quality of our touch is important.

John Naisbitt in his 1984 best selling book, *Megatrends*, states, "Whenever new technology is introduced into society, there must be a counterbalancing human response—that is, high touch, or the technology is rejected."[4] The more high technology around us the more the need for human touch.[5] Naisbitt is also talking about touch through social interaction, the need for more nurturing human, relationships, and creative outlets. High tech he concludes is responsible for the rise of the human potential and complementary health movements because, "we must learn to balance the material wonder of technology with the spiritual demands of our human nature."[6]

Hands Only

There is no reason for the use of tools in our work when we consider the anatomy of the foot and its sensitive periosteum. Trained, experienced hands can assess and evaluate, machines cannot. One excuse often given for the use of implements is that the practitioner's thumbs and fingers can become overworked. However, techniques properly applied using correct body postures will lessen this risk. It is also the practitioner's responsibility to see that his tools—his hands and body—are taken care of properly through massage and exercise. In addition, deep pressure is not needed as light touch can be more effective than heavy pressure. Nobel Prize winner Dr. Edgar Adrian showed that the electrical intensity of the nerve impulse depended on the size of the nerve rather than upon the strength of the stimulus.[7] However, light touch in our case, does not refer to energetic work, for one needs to go deeper than the surface layer of the skin to be effective. And most importantly, implements take away from touch and bring in more high tech. It is the touch our clients want to experience. It is the nurturing of the human touch our clients are in need of. It is the importance of the human touch we must

never lose sight of.

The effects of palpation are multi-dimensional, working on the physical and non-physical. In terms of healing different physiological processes come into play. At the start, when we palpate we stimulate the nervous system. Then the sympathetic nervous system reacts. By the end of a session the parasympathetic system responds and relaxation occurs. Relaxation of the foot will reverberate up the spinal column and through the autonomic nerve ganglia to the organs and other parts of the body due to the close ties between the central nervous system and the autonomic nervous system. The inclusion of the function of the brain stem and the role it plays in interpreting touch validates reflexognosy and the results achieved. The result of palpation to the receptors on the feet, coupled with joint activation, produces the range of reactions we see on the physical level. Stimulus travels at enormous speeds and involves very diverse areas of the body. Removal of articular lesions, coupled with hormonal activation, triggering an endocrine response, stimulation to the circulatory and lymphatic systems, and all nervous systems, makes reflexognosy a very powerful therapy.

The quality of touch is important to consider and in response, the practitioner of reflexognosy, uses only the hands. Tools and mechanical devices lessen the element of human touch and supports the impersonal nature of technology which is already rampant in our society. The lack of touch (on all levels) is partly the reason that society has become dissatisfied with traditional medicine. Let us not fall into the same trap. Reflexognosy, as a complementary health discipline, provides clients the opportunity to find wholistic health through the compensating factor of human touch.

In spite of our touch and best intentions, sometimes people do not heal and we take it personally asking, "Have I failed? Has reflexognosy failed as a therapy?" When this happens we need to assess what the nature of illness is and why is it that some people fail to respond.

---

[1] Rossi, Laurence and DavidCheek. *Mind-Body Therapy: Ideodynamic Healing in Hypnosis*, pg.214.

[2] Winsor, Henry M.D. The Medical Times, "Sympathethetic Segmental Distrubances—II", November 1921, pgs. 267-271.

[3] Ingham, Eunice. *Stories the Feet Can Tell*, pg. 2.

[4] Naisbitt, John. *Megatrends*, 1984, pg. 39

[5] Naisbitt, pg. 53.

[6] Naisbitt, pg. 40.

[7] Issel, Christine. *Reflexology: Art, Science & History*, pg. 33.

Chapter 13

The Nature of Illness

"Life as we know it demands disease; it is unthinkable without it. Disease becomes more than a blackish prelude to death. It becomes the harbinger of life."
—Larry Dossey

"Diseases may be cured, but people require healing, and those whose diseases may never be cured may still experience profound healing."
—Janet F. Quinn

While the last few chapters have been focusing very heavily on the physical aspect of the body and the role feet play in health, one could easily assume that health is the absence of disease or deviations from normalcy in function. However, this is not the entire picture. In order to comprehend why people become ill in the first place one must have an intricate knowledge of the complex regulatory systems of the human body as well as a greater awareness of the subtle vehicles of consciousness which interact with the physical form. The tissues which compose our physical form are fed not only by oxygen, glucose, and chemical nutrients, but also by higher vibrational energies through the chakras and meridians which endow the physical frame with the properties of life and creative expression. Within us we have all the healing require-

ments to heal our ills for the time allocated to us. We need to be aware of this and learn how to access it as part of our healing response.

There is Only One Disease: Congestion

Left brain logic will say: a symptom is a warning of a change in structure or function, and disease is a breakdown somewhere in the function of the structure. Acute disease is caused by a sudden traumatic condition while chronic disease develops slowly from prolonged malfunctioning or improper use. This is only part of the picture. Whether we look at the nature of illness from the purely physical or the energetic model, in essence there is only one disease and that is congestion, when functional dis-ease impairs the body's flow of physical and subtle energy, nutrients, blood supply, and oxygen.

All illness is congestive in nature which in turn causes a lack of balance within the body. The goal of reflexognosy is to assist the body in freeing up congestion and encourage balance, not to cure a specific symptom or disease. The reflexognosist will provide the techniques that are conducive to relaxation and assist the body to decongest providing the opportunity to achieve dynamic results.

Health and illness are not opposite ends of the spectrum. It is often impossible to draw a sharp division between health and illness. Both are part of us. Just like riding a bicycle, we cannot remain in a state of perfect balance. The systems in our body are moving, however unperceptively, back and forth, like our breath, to maintain balance. The entire system is designed to be self-regulating, which is why most imbalances correct themselves without effort, healing regularly. Outside intervention is only required for stubborn and persistent blockages. Physical disease may be assisted to balance by a positive mental attitude and social support so that the overall state is one of well-being, but this comes from within. On the other hand, emotional problems or social isolation can make a person feel sick in spite of physical fitness. Therefore, an overall discussion of health must encompass a multi-disciplinary study of human nature and also investigate the quality of one's existence and the role disease plays in our lives. If health were a simple matter of fixing or replacing malfunctioning parts everyone would be well.

Contrary to what is often thought, illness is not necessarily an enemy. It does not come to "punish us for our sins or transgressions", and we do not necessarily create the illness because of improper thoughts and actions. There is no need to dump guilt upon oneself when one becomes ill and question, "What did I do wrong?" Illness is an opportunity for growth and development. It can come as a teacher to aid us in a change of thought process and outlook on life. It can guide us to a deeper understanding of ourselves and our relationship to the world. It is a natural process. Without illness our body would not produce certain elements to keep us alive. Health, as well as disease, is about learning how to live; that is an educational process.

The question then arises, should we consider ourselves facilitators and educators if we are helping our clients find and restore balance and thus health in their lives? Dossey (1993) states, *"It is impossible in principle to make rigid, uniform connections between life events and physical illness."*[1] [emphasis Rogers & Issel] Dossey encourages the practitioner to ask clients, what meaning *they* place on their illness. This is very relevant; how the client interprets their illness will have a direct influence on outcome. [Here the term patient is purposely not used in reference to the client. Not that its use could be illegal, but we do not wish the client to receive the subliminal connotation to be a patient and passive. The person must be active in their own healing.]

In dealing with energy, one concentrates on the process—the concepts of flow, rhythm and mind/body connections. We need to ask, what happens in the process. The body has an enormous capacity and equipment to heal and rejuvenate itself given the opportunity to do so. But first the client must take responsibility for his/her own health by becoming committed and actively involved in the learning process.

Illness is the most constructive natural thing that happens to us. The healing power that can be created in our body from illness is enormous. Illness tells us how healthy we actually are. If you are sick and can get well then you know how much healing energy you have. If you were never sick your system would not produce the healing power illness stimulates, nor promote an awareness for your body pertaining to its needs. It points us in the direction of what system of our body cannot cope with certain stimuli and needs to be supported with additional nutrients or perhaps loving care. The needs of our body are simple: food, air, water, communication, and non-invasive touch as foundational needs. In acute illness or trauma there may be times surgical intervention will be needed. This is part of the process and complementary disciplines can provide support and enhance the healing process.

As people wanting to help humanity, reflexognosists must not be under the illusion that they can ever abolish illness or make a person well. Illness is in our nature. If we feel a bit despondent, depressed, invariably we are going to get sick because it is in our nature to react that way. This tells us that the emotions and psychological states are very much linked. So the state of our mind influences the state of our health. Our body recovers from so many illnesses in our lifetime, it is a remarkable healing unit.

It is important to remember that illness can originate at many levels of our multidimensional being and not just at the level of the physical body. Although there are many external agents of disease—bacteria, viruses, environmental toxins and carcinogens—they are less likely to adversely affect the body of an individual who is in good physical and mental health. An understanding of subtle energy can have beneficial effects upon emotional and physical diseases. The fact that our consciousness can influence the energy fields has important implication for both medicine and psychology.

Our emotions lead us in and out of the cycle of change from illness to well being. When we are dealing with human beings we need to be aware that the emotions are triggering this cycle, it is not some physiological breakdown like Western medicine views the body. Emotional reactions in the body upset the balance and may produce physiological symptoms. We would, as natural therapists, observe the body wholistically. It is the emotions that play a role that will lead people in and out of illness to well-being and well-being back to illness. So when we look at people we must consider their emotional state. This is why we need to think critically about the aspect of touch. When we are touching people we are dealing with very deep-seated emotions. We must never judge a person's thoughts or experiences. Everyone is different. Interpreting a body type or analyzing parts of a body and evaluating their deep emotional thoughts or experiences is an invasion of the client's privacy. These people fall outside of any profession and have no foundation for their judgmental claims. All people are complete beings with their *own* personal experiences.

Just as we have models to follow in complementary medicine we also have at least one model in the body-mind connection and health. In modern psychotherapy the therapeutic process is not seen as a treatment of disease but as a journey in self-exploration and non-rational outcomes as valid. The therapist becomes the facilitator of a 'process' in which the client bears full responsibility. The therapist creates an environment conducive to self-explorations and acts as a guide while the process unfolds. To assume such a role a psychotherapist needs qualities such as warmth and genuineness, the ability to listen and to show empathy, the ability to withhold judgment and promote unconditional understanding and acceptance. In addition, the therapist's own stage of personal development is vital. This approach requires not only some basic knowledge of human biology, psychology and social sciences, but also experience, wisdom, compassion, and concern for the patient as a human being. A paradox occurs with this model.

Webster's Dictionary defines 'a paradox' as a statement that seems contradictory, unbelievable, or absurd, but that may be true in fact.[2] Dossey (1993), explains the paradox by pointing out that society has conditioned us to think that those healing strategies that employ 'doing' seem reasonable. They make sense and can be explained by science. 'Doing' approaches are usually invasive therapies and include such things as surgery, drugs, exercise and diet. On the other hand, 'being' therapies, lacking reasonable explanations, appear to be irrational. The results of generally non-invasive approaches such as counseling, prayer and imagery, more often than not, happen without reason and could be classified as the placebo effect or miracles. But the body and 'being' therapies contain a mysterious element. Miracles do not always happen. If they did a formula would be discovered to bring about a predictable result and bring the 'being' therapy into the 'doing' category. But when healing does occur it is usually accompanied by a paradoxical realization that there is an importance to illness and that life without it may not be desirable.[3]

We need to acknowledge that healing is mysterious, beyond our control and manipulation, yet open to our conscious participation and intention. According to Dr. O. Carl Simonton of the Simonton Cancer Center, the most health-supporting emotional state seems not to be enthusiasm or even optimism, but serenity and peacefulness on the part of the client and the practitioner.

Treatment of disease and illness is the domain of the medical profession. As reflexognosists we do not need to look for symptomology. What we need to look for is systemology. In other words, what is the weak system that is presenting in this person's body? What pressure, to what system, and why is the pressure there? Linking biomechanics and congestion leads to constructive answers. We will avoid making references to specific symptomologies or diseases. Instead of thinking a client has PMS, we will think she has a female reproductive system imbalance that is congestive in nature and evaluate in a caring partnership what needs are to be met by the inclusion of reflexognosy.

Fear

Fear is one of the greatest problems associated with illness and can hamper the healing process. "Fear is a poison that can affect every part of the human organism," wrote Eunice Ingham in 1951. She continues: "The power of thought can make us live or die. Yes, the power of our thoughts can make us live a happy and healthy life, or fill our body with poison, resulting in pain and disease. ...We can really invite disaster by our negative fear and thoughts and bring about many a serious condition from the effect these negative thoughts will have on the functioning of our glands, changing the normal metabolic balance."[4]

Most people are frightened about what is going to happen to them. However, we can approach fear with the Buddhist theory on crisis. Crisis is two sided: it produces fear *and* opportunity. Out of something that is bad comes something good. We owe it to ourselves to stick with the subject that created fear, which, to quote an old adage, defines fear as:

False
Evidence
Appearing
Real.

People respond not only to physical reality, but also to their thoughts, memories, plans, symbols, emotions, etc. We respond fully to nonphysical events as if they were physically dangerous, or physically non-threatening. Our response to a situation either engages the sympathetic or parasympathetic nervous system: we are either relaxed or stressed. Most disease and tension is caused by fear arising unconsciously from the activity of the sympathetic nervous system. Fear can make us sick without our realizing it.

We need to continue to examine fear from all angles, and in turn we will produce the necessary change. We have the opportunity to help our clients to do likewise. In helping them discover their fears and examining them from different angles, we can assist them to change, which in turn, will produce different emotions and growth making the symptoms unnecessary. This compliments Dr. Larry Dossey's advice by placing meaning to the subject, and looking at the 'person' not the condition.

The Nature of Healing

The human mind, not the physician, was placed in charge of managing our health. The brain can be seen as a computer, while the mind is the computer programmer. Health maintenance is one of the primary functions of the mind. Psychological and social factors interpreted by the mind can influence our immunity to infectious and other diseases. The mind transforms thought, feelings and beliefs into chemical messages and our cells change their activity in response to such messages from our mind and others. The mind interprets and translates the complex changes in our environment. The heart itself does not perceive that a work situation is unbearable. The immune system does not know whether its owner just lost a job or a spouse. Neither does the brain. Health is influenced by the stability of our social worlds, mental and emotional lives and internal physiology.

Healing is the unification and alignment of the body/mind/spirit and occurs with the removal of obstructions to the body's own inherent wisdom to seek balance. It has little to do with curing of symptoms and ailments. It is a process rather than an event and involves growth and development. As Deepak Chopra said, "I think the answer is that all medicine works by helping a patient live through his disease, moment by moment, until the balance swings away from sickness toward cure."[5]

Though it would be overly simplistic to say that the mind causes or cures illness, it is clear that our emotions, attitudes, and beliefs can influence our health and that altering thoughts and emotions can have a powerful effect on health as well. For reflexognosists, as well as those receiving the session, the lesson is clear; the two most important allies the reflexognosist has are: the client and the client's mind. Our responsibility and role in the health of our client must always be taken with the utmost seriousness. Seriousness does not mean with a lack of humor however, because humor in clinical practice is an integral component in healing. Humor is in opposition to anger and depression. Seriousness involves a deep respect and reverence for the other person and a humility within ourselves, for truly we are not the healer—the multi-dimensional nature of the client is.

Remember the therapist is the one who interacts with the client whilst nature [or the client] does the healing.

Relaxation and Immune Strengthening

Research has proven that the right precondition for the healing of any disorder is the strengthening of the immune system. The principle technique for this is relaxation. The relaxation response was described extensively by Herbert Benson (1975) and it refers to a psychophysiological state in which the parasympathetic nervous system is activated. This effects a balance with the sympathetic nervous system and allows for the body to engage in restorative patterns. Deepak Chopra concurs. In Ayurvedic medicine, a level of total, deep relaxation is the most important precondition for curing any disorder. Reflexognosy is one way to activate the relaxation response. Touch through reflexognosy allows the integration of the physical and mental/emotional bodies which is often accompanied by reduction or elimination of pain for a length of time. This affect of reflexognosy gives the client a glimpse of what life can be like without their illness. Hand contact also supports the metabolic demands of regeneration through circulatory and electromagnetic stimulation. Adding to this interchange, a less stressful gait pattern will provide a firm foundation to healing.

What is required for this subtle form of self-regulation to work is not control but a state of deep relaxation in which all control is relinquished. In such a state, channels of communication between the conscious and the unconscious mind open up and facilitate the integration of psychological and biological functions. Due to this integration of body and mind, often during the course of a session, reflexognosists will find a client discussing events that he or she did not consciously know was troubling him or her or would not be willing to discuss under normal circumstances. Rossi and Cheek (1994) may provide us with a reason why this occurs. "The memories of these traumatic events are said to be deeply imprinted as physiological memory, tissue memory, or muscle memory. We propose that all these designations are actually metaphors for the special state-dependent encoding of memories by the stress released hormonal information substances." [6]

Think for a moment about how your feet feel when you are under stress or when you are exposed to major shock or trauma. The toes curl or extend stressing the intricate musculature. This musculature houses a memory as indicated above. Palpation of this musculature may be the reason why certain clients have emotional responses, such as tears, during a session. This is not to imply that all clients will behave in this manner but it is a valid explanation for the times it does. Release of the tension in the area releases the memory that produced the physical reaction in the first place.

Reflexognosists do not think the discipline effects only the physical body, therefore, as tactile practitioners, our role goes beyond simply being a technician to one of being an educator and counselor.

To integrate the physical and psychological therapies into reflexognosy makes it a wholistic discipline. A small shift in thought process and an extension of existing ideas, is all that is required since most practitioners recognize an interdependence of mind and body in health and illness. There is a need to develop communication skills. We must know where the client is in their personal development—what state of mind, what changes are occurring in the client's life, how the client responds to work, family and friends. To be wholistic practitioners, as reflexognosists, we need to be concerned with knowing, not so much about the disease, but knowing more about the person whose body is battling the disease process.

Healing is stimulated via the *function* of the body. This is total function, all parts working in harmony. Function will be affected by structure, particularly if there is a deviation from normalcy within a structure. The stimulus to the body's functional components produces the healing. Reflexognosy blends both function and deviation.

The future of healing will involve the formulation of new conceptual models, the expansion of existing educational programs or the development of new ones. An educational program presenting a multi-disciplinary study of human nature and health will be invaluable for a wholistic approach to our clients. To understand the models of 'energy medicine' scientifically, it would seem that one would concentrate on the process—the concepts of flow, rhythm, mind/body connections—and the soul/spirit concept in healing as part of their philosophical base. These new conceptual models are applied in reflexognosy.

This expanded view of health and healing, the study of anatomy and physiology through systems, subtle energy, anatomy of the leg and foot, and the focus on the feet themselves are all part of core subjects for the profession of reflexognosy. The time spent working on the feet gives us valuable information, that if channeled correctly, creates a powerful and unique healthcare profession.

Reflexognosy will not amount to a major revolution, but a shift in thought process since most practitioners already recognize the interdependence of mind and body in health and illness and therefore are already involved with the major shift in paradigm occurring in the emerging health care system.

Above all else, we must as human beings search for happiness; this quest will lead to quality living—quantity is not the issue.

Remember: "Living is a sexually transmitted, terminal condition, the fact we are living means we will die, therefore, enjoy the journey and the process." —Sandi Rogers

[1] Dossey, Larry. *Meaning Medicine*, pg. 15.

[2] *Webster's Dictionary*, pg. 979.

[3] Dossey, pg. 204-212.

[4] Ingham, Eunice, *Stories the Feet Have Told*, pg., 39.

[5] Chopra, Deepak, *Quantum Healing*, Bantam Books, New York, 1990, pg. 212.

[6] Rossi, Laurence and DavidCheek. *Mind-Body Therapy: Ideodynamic Healing in Hypnosis*, WW Norton, New York, 1994, pg.214.

Chapter 14

Professional Considerations for the New Paradigm

"Love itself, I found, is not enough to be truly therapeutic; you have to understand what you are doing, you have to act knowledgeably."

—Dolores Krieger

The first question we can ask is: What is a discipline? Then, what is a profession? Next, what is the difference between a discipline and a profession? And finally, how is a profession created?

A discipline is an area of knowledge and theory that can exist purely for itself, but a profession must have a practical application. The primary object of a discipline is to gain knowledge while in a profession it is to apply knowledge in a way that serves others; the integration of the theoretical with the practical.

Abraham Flexner created the first set of criteria for professional status in 1915. Today, his criteria are still the most commonly accepted. Flexner identified six characteristics that determine whether a field of study is a profession. These are:

1. Intellectual activity or a body of knowledge—while physical skills may be involved in performing the work, it must have an intellectual base.

2. Practical use—even though it has an intellectual base, that knowledge has no value unless it is applied.

3. Research which clarifies and validates anecdotal claims and results in new knowledge and ideas.

4. Self-organization—a profession has formal organizations which facilitate communication.

5. The capacity for communication—both externally and internally with its members which enables them to work together to solve common problems and distribute information and raise professional standards through educational requirements.

6. Dedication to helping others—a profession exists, in part, to help

improve the lives of other people.[1]

Seventy-five years later Appelbaum and Lawton (1990) in *Ethics and the Professions*, describe a profession in much the same way. "A profession consists of a group of people organized to serve a body of specialized knowledge in the interests of society."[2] New groups emerge as work and information grow more specialized and a well defined training is put in place. In addition, "Each profession maintains standards of excellence, oversees work performance, and trains new members. Each shares a professional vocabulary, usually not understood by the lay person. Each provides a means of professional communications [in the form of journals and meetings]. And, each has its professional code of ethics which specifies the moral consideration of professional life as well as penalties and sanctions for violating them."[3] Two other important additions to this list would be protecting the public by having a system to deal with complaints which encompasses, the question of governmental or self-regulation; and of course, a clientele that needs and demands the services of the field.

Standards of Excellence

Standards of excellence in education and training are the foundation upon which a profession is built and the safety of the public is assured. Without standards there is no way to measure performance, conduct research, develop well defined training and acquire a consistent professional vocabulary with which to communicate between each other and with other health care profes-

sionals. A professional vocabulary is not for elitist purposes but to avoid ambiguities and confusion.

It is the purpose of reflexognosy to be a wholistic discipline. Just as the Newtonian paradigm of physics was extended by quantum physics, the principles of reflexognosy go beyond the limited views of some already established disciplines. With new knowledge, comprehension of the multi-dimensional nature of the work and its effects, reflexognosy can make a significant contribution to healthcare.

Reflexognosists are seeking to manage health and illness and are looking to the feet. Eunice Ingham's call for new developments has been answered in reflexognosy. Reflexognosy deals directly with the chemistry and structure of the physical body through tactile stimulation and then goes beyond this to a world of subtle energy and wholistic management. It deals with energy that can be strongly influenced by the mental and emotional activity of individuals. Therefore, reflexognosy works on the four levels of man—emotionally, mentally, spiritually, and physically, although, as yet, some of these levels are not clearly defined.

The National College of Traditional Medicine in Melbourne, Australia offers advanced training courses in reflexognosy. Courses are taught internationally as well. For the person wishing to enter a field of training with high educational and professional standards consistent with other professions that encompasses a focus toward whole health management, reflexognosy offers this. The goal is for its practitioners to be seen as professional foot assessors who, on one level, work to improve the biomechanical function of the feet and to assist in health. It involves the application of appropriate pressure to the legs and feet by the hands of a trained practitioner to facilitate a healing response through physiological and psychological changes in the body. Physiological, by increased circulation, lymphatic flow, nerve response to the receptors of the feet, proprioceptors, sensory receptors, and extroceptors. Psychological, through the release of emotions and flow of energy. This is the genesis of an entirely new profession that blends the trilogy of subtle energies, anatomy and structural alignment of the body to facilitate well-being. The practitioner and the modality call upon extensive knowledge of the function of anatomy and physiology, biomechanics of the leg and foot, soft tissue management and draws conclusions from professional assessment of the feet. Observations are made to detail structural deviation from normalcy and evaluates elementary foot pathologies.

Reflexognosy provides hands-on skills to release tension and promote a more structurally balanced pedal foundation, resulting in a less rigid body. An extension of this would be found in a healthier circulatory system. Clinical results have proven to be very favorable with the discipline. Reflexognosy provides a direct affect to the peripheral vascular return; and better health as a result of improved circulation.

Professional Considerations for Reflexognosy

Reflexognosy demands high levels of educational standards and a wider curriculum as well as more in-clusive ethical considerations.

The education of the professional foot assessor must be concerned with the development of a critically aware frame of mind, not with the uncritical assimilation of previously defined skills or bodies of knowledge. Critical reflection promotes healthy skepticism. The principles of praxis can be used to aid a paradigm shift.[4] Praxis is the accepted practice or custom of an art or skill. It comes from the Greek word *prasso* meaning to do. The praxis process involves:

- Learners becoming acquainted with skills

- Students applying these in real life settings

- Practitioners then reflecting with other learners on their experiences in these settings

- In turn, redefining how these skills might be altered by context

- Students then reapplying the altered ones in other real life settings which begins the process over again.[5]

It is important that prior to forming an opinion we evaluate the concept from every point of view. We apply critical thinking skills and constantly ask questions and call for discussion about each and every facet of the therapy. We must look for definitions for each word that is used. This process is exciting and stimulating. The outcome would be to develop a new consciousness, promote attitudinal shifts and encourage explanation of the subjects.

169

Brookfield believes critical thinking, comprised of the processes of identifying and challenging assumptions, and imagining and exploring alternatives, is an indication of an open and healthy society. The authors strongly encourage the use of critical thinking skills in the development of reflexognosy as a profession.

Educational Standards

There is a wealth of knowledge throughout the world that bears relevance to the educational needs of reflexognosists and it is time that all the literature be pooled to strengthen the skills of the profession. At the same time, reflexognosy must develop from a firm foundation. In order that a proper foundation can be built, reflexognosy must, like most other therapies, base its philosophy upon science, both social and anthropological. This can be achieved through education and training of practitioners to the highest level possible. The subjects included in an educational program must be adapted to suit the needs of the profession. For instance, as reflexognosists work in hospitals with acute cases, or in private practice with chronic cases, though not mutually exclusive, two different educational needs immerge.

Standards play a major role in assessment. Standards provides the opportunity to develop our profession and promote dialogue between professionals. There is a need for a definitive language to aid communication in teaching and research.

A wholistic interpretation of the body via the feet has sound scientific validation endorsed by research that has followed correct protocol. However, both hard science and case histories are required to create a balance for the profession. To quote an old axiom, "Practice without theory is like sailing an uncharted sea. Theory without practice is like not going to sea at all." Reflexognosy cannot be all theory and no hands-on techniques, nor can it be all hands-on without understanding the body, its structure and function, theories and philosophies, and the dynamics of healing.

Training in critical thinking, discernment, understanding data, perceiving relations, elaborating concepts, formulating principles and making evaluations, are all necessary for the reflexognosist. The raw data taken into the mind is information. Learning is the knowledge gained by study and experience. Generally in higher education these concepts are applied to the humanities rather than to science and technology. But it is the belief of the authors that in order to have knowledge, the practitioner must be well informed in their subject, having investigated it from every point of view. Curriculum development for the reflexognosist will be broad. For it is the purpose of reflexognosy to go beyond the limited views of any one therapy. With new knowledge, comprehension of the multi-dimensional nature of man, the work and its effects, reflexognosy can make a significant contribution to wellness and healthcare in whatever setting it is practiced.

Ethics

A profession establishes a sytem of values through a code of ethics which specifies the moral consideration of professional life as well as penalties and sanctions for violating them. Probably the most commonly known concept of ethics is the Hippocratic oath which begins with the charge to do no harm.

All who work with people in an intimate way develop a unique relationship with their clients which is part of the healing process. Beyond written rules, ethical principles guide our attitude toward life in general. Ethics is concerned with moral behavior. Personal morals are expressions of a person's subjective beliefs and religious and cultural background. Ethics, on the other hand, do not look at morals in the strictest religious sense, but in the broader view of ethical behavior as being an attitude of reverence for life. This reverence includes an appreciation and respect for the being of the client and all others whom we meet in life, and a respect for the powerful healing modality reflexognosy is. While reflexognosy is a non-invasive physical therapy, the practitioner must be non-invasive on all levels. This involves a regard for boundaries in the following ways:

- Total respect for a client's subtle energy space. During and for some time after a session, a client is in a state of enhanced suggestibility. Therefore the practitioner must be careful in his intent, language or any suggestions made as we may be setting up a response in the body.

- Viewing your clients as 'beings' rather than a disease or diagnosis and respecting the right of the clients to self-determine their course of treatment and amount of wellness they wish to attain.

- Total respect for client confidentiality including the process and pace through which the client is moving, whenever or whatever emotions or thoughts surface, treating them with a non-judgmental attitude. This includes not looking at part of the anatomy and making judgments.

- Encouragement in the client's sense of self-confidence and personal power, not in you as a healer. Every practitioner must be willing to explore their own motivations and avoid setting up a co-dependency situation.

- A respect and knowledge for the contraindications and cautions in reflexognosy.

- An acknowledgment of the need for your own intellectual, personal and spiritual development.

Respecting boundaries provides a safe environment that brings forth positive, life-enhancing outcomes which are not controlled by either the client or the practitioner.

In dealing with questions of ethics we need to retain a sense of the process and development in the field as well as the means of evaluating and analyzing decisions. We also need to remember all questions regarding ethics are subject to on-going debate. The key in ethics is to explore what, how, and why, we do what we do with the needs of both the reflexognosist and the client included in any objective analysis and discussion.

Ethical decisions are group standards based on value-laden input from those within the field insofar as they call forth decisions and judgments regarding the:

1. Practice

2. Method

3. Policy and

4. Research of a group of members within a profession.

Questions of ethics are never answered "once and for all". A single new input can change a belief in what the right action is. Therefore in regard to ethics it is important to keep communication open within a profession so that disagreements can be aired and hopefully resolved with people agreeing to disagree. According to Appelbaum & Lawton (1990), the answers to ethical questions will be found by discovering what is morally acceptable to do using as objective reasoning and critical thinking as possible. "An ethical theory thus serves to articulate the duties, responsibilities, and obligations that affect what we ought to do. The virtues of an ethical theory, as opposed to our ordinary feelings, opinions and beliefs, lie in its being coherent and complete."[6]

Through various codes of ethics employed in the health field, such issues as patient/client relationship, confidentiality, informed consent, honesty through full and fair disclosure of services, referral to a primary care physician, and other ethical questions are dealt with. Within a discipline, before one can fully and fairly disclose their therapy, they must have an understanding as to their scope of practice and how the discipline works. Expected outcomes in relation to the discipline must also

be conveyed to the client. This information provides the client data from which to grant an informed consent for treatment. Consent can be given verbally or in writing. The establishment of a Code of Ethics helps to ensure public safety and builds a strong foundation for a field by setting professional boundaries.

Contraindications

The discussion of professional boundaries brings us next to the controversial subject of contraindications. There is no panacea for all ills—reflexognosists must be aware of their limitations via contraindications. When discussing contraindications they need to be examined in a scientific fashion in the light of the most current knowledge of anatomy and physiology, and secondly from a reflexognosy perspective. In science, for every action there is an equal and opposite reaction. Therefore, if reflexognosy is producing an action, one is going to get a reaction. Reflexognosists must not let their caring attitude interfere with effectively caring for clients. They must recognize the limitations and consequences of reflexognosy.

As the acceptance of reflexognosy grows, reflexognosists will see more and more people who have serious health problems but choose not to seek conventional medicine treatment first, or during their illness but prefer to assume responsibility for their own treatment program. In these days of litigation, reflexognosists must be absolutely professional in everything they do, including being mindful of contraindications, making referrals to primary health care practitioners and in some cases, refusing to work on a client for their own health's sake, and referring the client to an appropriate practitioner.

Certain issues arise when we speak of contraindication. Contraindications are the basis of our:

1. Awareness of the outcomes we reach

2. Effectiveness of therapy

3. Ethics

4. Client protection on all levels—physical, emotional, mental and spiritual

5. Legal safety for both the client and practitioner

There are three words that form the basis of this discussion: caution, contraindication, and precaution. Let us look at each of the words that have entered the field in reference to contraindications.

Turning to *The New Elizabethan Reference Dictionary and The New Standard Illustrated Dictionary* we find '*caution*' means 'to take heed; to care to avoid injury'. We must surely act with caution each and every minute in clinical practice. Therefore, this word must be in our vocabulary and adhered to with every client/patient we see.

Contraindication means: 'a symptom which is adverse to the usual care and techniques; it dictates a different or contrary approach than usual.' This word fits with the medical model and clearly is suitable to consider where we are dealing with clients and health.

Precaution means: 'prudent foresight; a measure taken beforehand, to guard against or bring about

something; to caution or warn beforehand; to give warning to.' Does this fit with a model that we could use? It is the authors' view that it does not. We need to use the terms caution and contraindication instead. We, as professionals, will use caution each time we see a client and abide by contraindications when needed.

In relation to contraindications we would propose there are two types: *Relative* and *Absolute*. A *relative contraindication* is where you will choose another therapy or choose another part of the body to work on. An *absolute contraindication* is where no therapy is recommended for the time **the condition is present** unless clearance is obtained from the attending physician first. For instance:

1. When there is a **physical trauma** to the feet, where touch is too painful, maybe you would work on the hand or above the foot and do the leg. This is a *relative contraindication*.

2. When there is a **recent fracture** or break in the bones of the foot, this is another case of *relative contraindication*. Although painful, it would also be possible that a hairline fracture could become an actual break if the application of pressure is used, so alternative treatment is required.

3. **Tinea** is a contraindication as it is contagious. However, podiatrists are currently debating whether tinea is contagious. But until there is more research on the matter and podiatry agrees on this subject, it should be avoided. It is an *absolute contraindication*.

173

4. **Dry scaly skin** condition of which you, the practitioner, is unsure of its pathology. *Absolute contraindication* is warranted until the pathology is determined.

5. **Certain medical complications** are an *absolute contraindication.* A client/patient who has recently suffered a **stroke** and is under medical supervision for the possibility of additional strokes or diagnosed with a blood clot, should lead the practitioner to conclude, that until a release is given by the consulting physician, do not proceed. This is an absolute contraindication as stimulation to the circulatory system could be dangerous. This also applies to **certain forms of cancer**, notably lymphomas where the primary care physician has prescribed medication to slow the circulation or lymph flow. Cancer sufferers, once authorized by the attending physician to receive reflexognosy, may benefit greatly. **Heart attack** and **organ transplant** patients also fall under this category. Other medical conditions include **diabetes** or **unstable blood pressure**. The application of reflexognosy influences blood pressure and blood sugar levels. It is important blood pressure be stabilized first without the influence of reflexognosy. The same is true of diabetes and the use of insulin. Once the condition is stabilized then the use of reflexognosy becomes a *caution* with the client and his or her attending physician monitoring drug dosage. Due to their unknown synergistic effect amongst themselves and with reflexognosy those clients with heavy prescription drug use would also be an **absolute contraindication**.

6. Another *absolute contraindication* is the **first trimester of pregnancy** because it is the most unpredictable time. We stimulate acupressure points and some of the most powerful stimulators are located around the ankles— Spleen 6 and the descending meridians, gallbladder 40 and bladder 60. Oriental practitioners warn these points could induce miscarriage and therefore they avoid working on them.

7. **Neuroma,** or nerve entrapment in the foot, is *an absolute contraindication* until the condition is managed by a consulting podiatrist with anti-inflammatories and the nerve is no longer entrapped.

8. **Infections** are a *relative contraindication.* The professional will consider location and grade of the infection before commencing a session.

9. A **psychologically disturbed** person is a *relative contraindication.* Touch can bring up unresolved issues which the reflexognosist may not be trained to deal with. Unless specifically trained in this area, the professional will acknowledge the limit of his or her training, scope of practice and licensing.

10. The **amount of pressure** is a *caution.* Common sense dictates lighter pressure be used:

• When you see a client for the first time.

- When acute or chronic pain is present. Nothing settles pain and anguish better than a foot session.

- When there is swelling or puffiness around the legs and feet.

- When the client is obviously old with delicate bone structure. Heavy pressure on such an individual could conceivably cause bruising so extra care must be taken.

- When treating a young child who's skin is delicate and whose bones are forming.

The foot has a direct link physiologically with the rest of the body and the subtle energy systems. As we develop more knowledge about reflexognosy through research, and it is recorded for scientific scrutiny, we will be in a better position to ascertain which category certain conditions will fall under and whether they will be relative or absolute contraindications. A professional will proceed with absolute caution and assess each situation fully and then select an appropriate treatment drawing from a broad knowledge base. For instance, it may be decided that deeper pressure can be applied because the client, exhibiting good structure, has had at least one prior session with no negative reaction

The motto of reflexognosy is: 'First care, then learning'. The reflexognosist will always have a caring attitude in mind first, even before engaging in the learning process and seeing a client. If we do not have a caring outlook, the rest—observing the client, assessment, and the application of tactile skills—is futile.

Tactile Skills

Basic reflexognosy skills include the development of tactile sensitivity within the practitioner. This skill is fundamental to the documentation of the client's progress, especially when referral to another practitioner is warranted.

The development of a tactile sense takes time and practice. The experienced reflexognosist can detect changes in texture, color, contour, temperature and moisture of the skin surface. The practitioner can palpate through the subcutaneous tissue to detect changes in the quality of the superficial and deep tissue layers. Their training enables them to detect subtle changes in the range of motion pertaining to the joints.

According to osteopath Myron Beal (1967), palpation consists of three steps:

1. reception or sensing

2. transmission of sensory impulses

3. interpretation[7]

Reception is the process whereby stimuli are perceived by the tactile receptors of the fingers and the proprioceptors of the deep muscles and tendons. Reception is qualified by the experience of the examiner, the conditions of the examiner's hands [calluses interfere with tactile sensing], and the state of relaxation of the examiner. Tension results in contracted musculature, which produces excessive stimulation from the examiner's own muscle and tendon proprioceptors and causes interference with reception.

Transmission of the sensory impulses is the next step in palpation.

Interference with transmission may be caused by excessive proprioceptive stimulation on the examiner's part, created by awkward positions, excessive movement, or an inability to relax. There may be a dysfunction in the examiner's nervous system, which could interfere with sensory transmission. Hence the need for practice in order to relax so this inference can be minimized.

Interpretation is the final step in the palpatory experience. It consists of the perception and analysis of the impulses sent to the brain. Conscious attention and awareness are needed for the best reception. Interpretation is a process that is unique to each individual. It is based on experience and previous associations. It may be qualified by the reception of other sensory stimulation such as sight, sound or smell. Excessive tension on the examiner's part, loss of attention, preconceptions of what should be experienced and lack of experience in palpation, may all contribute to interference with the interpretive step of palpation.

Gross Anatomy

As foot therapy practitioners around the world go through the process of government recognition, their basic educational curriculum is being examined, challenged and subsequently expanded. Currently the South African government wants to require them to meet the same standards in science as the first two years of medical school. The corresponding requirements both chiropractors and homeopaths are required to complete. This includes taking anatomy with a lab involving cadavers. Is there a danger that, through this process,

our discipline loses 'art' and 'heart' and becomes more medically orientated? That the body becomes reduced to anatomical language, dehumanized or materialized? The emotional knee-jerk reaction to these questions by most practitioners is probably, yes. Especially for those of us who do not want to practice in the medical model. Once again, before we condemn something let's move away from emotions by applying our critical thinking skills.

The anatomy lab adds a dimension to the study of anatomy that takes the study of the human body from being an intellectual exercise only, to one involving the other senses. The student *feels* the shapes and textures of skin and bone, muscles and tendons, nerve and blood vessels; *sees* the colors and densities of the tissues, pathologies; *smells* the formaldehyde; *hears* the tearing of adhesions and the sawing or cracking of the bones in the most detailed courses. This is an important teaching method that helps the student who is a kinetic learner.

Furthermore, the human anatomy lab allows for a specialized kind of touch, one that destroys in order to promote understanding. Destroy it must, however, as students separate structures and trace them through various tissues, they actually physically see the interrelatedness of the body. Over and over they appreciate the body and express their wonder and awe. In anatomical language, 'reflection' is the physical turning back of large structures, such as skin flaps or muscles, so that the underlying parts can be seen. In the more conventional sense of the word, through reflection on the understanding that comes from this kind of anatomy class there often is an accompanying extension of the students' education into spiritual, philosophical and emotional dimensions. It is hard to see the cadaver without remembering that at one time it was a living being and speculating on what the person's life was like, what the experiences were and why he or she would have wanted to donate their body to science.

Interestingly it is reported that by the end of the course another dimension uncovered in the students is that they come to recognize and appreciate the gift of the cadavers. Legally in the US all cadavers are provided only through planned agreements by those who have made such a conscious choice. The fact that the cadaver has bequeathed her or his human form indicates that a choice was made in life for the enrichment of others. This gift students come to honor and it helps them to develop technical understanding without losing the human wisdom that will also be a part of his or her ability to work with clients.

A physical education major in US universities is required to take anatomy and physiology courses as well as kinesiology class with human anatomy labs. "Through my anatomy lab I gained a greater respect for the design of the human body. I was in awe of how complicated the body is. It was fascinating to see how ligaments are actually connected, the size and relationship of tissues, to feel how thick certain tissues are and the different layers, or the difference between arteries and veins, and to see distinct muscles. I was impressed by the uniqueness of body abnormalities in the different cadavers—we aren't all alike. It was interesting to actually

see pathologies. In a way it made learning the names of structures easier—I could remember and understand things better as I felt what was being studied. An anatomy lab with human cadavers makes the study of anatomy practical and real. It aided me in understanding and appreciating the human body so much more. The dead taught us, the living, how to touch," reports one student.

After completing a human anatomy lab students move on in life with a much better sense of what the human body contains. They appreciate its physical complexity with knowledge that is both more technical and in-depth which leads to a greater respect and sense of awe for the multi-dimensional aspects of our nature. To include gross anatomy in a reflexognosy curriculum at the university level may not be such a bad idea.

Communication Skills

When curriculums are under discussion, the need for communication skills is almost always a topic that comes up. The capacity for communication—both externally and internally is one of the previously mentioned hallmarks of a profession. The need for a definitive language to aid in communication is essential for teaching, research and dialogue with other professions.

A professional reflexognosist will converse with peers using anatomical terms. Anatomical terms are not medical terms, but the universal language all professionals use when referring to the body and its movements. One of the noticeable differences in reflexognosy training is the lack of charts as the practitioner learns the anatomy of the foot and when discussing an area of sensitivity identifies it in anatomical terms.

Many adjectives have been used by osteopathic physicians over the years to give meaning to palpatory observations. Some of the adjectives that are commonly used include:

- fixed versus non-fixed

- superficial versus deep

- soft versus hard

- hot versus cold

- painful versus non-painful

- rough versus smooth

- circumscribed versus diffuse

- compressible versus rigid

- flaccid versus firm

- pliable versus tight

- acute versus chronic[8]

Additional terms used by the reflexognosist will include those of the subtle energy medicines and other complementary therapies.

Beyond professional terminology further development of interpersonable communication skills with our colleagues and clients are required. Within the profession writing skills are needed for client documentations and referrals.

SOAP Notes

SOAP notes are used in the physical therapy and sports medicine fields when performing an examination and documenting client visits.

SOAP is an acronym meaning:

S = Subjective Examination—taking a client history which includes quoting the client as to his/her perception of a condition and/or the state of their health.

O = Objective Examination—by the practitioner noting visual observations, palpation findings, performing range of motion test.

A = Assessment—based on the subjective and objective findings conclusions are reached about the client's current state and how to proceed.

P = Plan—how you will proceed with the client. What exercises are to be given? How often will the client need to return? Is a referral warranted to another healthcare professional?

The use of SOAP notes are taught as part of the business skills portion of a curriculum.

Interpersonal Communication

Communication skills with clients will focus on non-verbal and verbal techniques of interaction and the development of self. The emotional aspect of the work and the dying process will be covered.

The Helping Relationship

Some think to go into this area is out of the scope of practice. The client should be referred to a psychologist or other trained counselor. One of the developments in our technical oriented society was been the professionalization of the helping process. The idea of helping, in the formal sense of counseling, is largely an American white middle-class phenomenon. In most other cultures, helping a person usually occurs in an informal setting, such as within families.[9]

To protect the public, helping functions over the years became limited to specialists with special education and credentials. However, as Brammer (1988) points out, "Helping is a function of *all* concerned human beings and is *not* limited to professional helpers." And that includes reflexognosists.

Others see communication skills as the art of active listening and something the reflexognosist should be trained in doing properly simply because our clients talk to us. More importantly when faced with emotional outpourings from a client, the practitioner must understand basic approaches in dealing with the client's psychological state.

As noted earlier, communication skills cover a wide variety of topics and includes the body/mind connection. Therefore, in a communication skills course the following questions and topics can be included:

- What does it mean to communicate? A fundamental problem in all human relations is our difficulty in reaching one another successfully, what are the secrets of doing so? What is communicated through physical touch, through voice, through posture and gestures?

- How much verbalizing, on the part of the practitioner and client should there be during a session?

- Helping, what does it mean? Doing anything for other people without their consent frequently is manipulative and often is destructive. Even when the help is solicited and given with the best of intentions, it may have an unplanned detrimental effect on the client.

- In the broadest sense it means to help normal individuals function at a higher level, but what does it mean to the individual reflexognosist personally? How does he or she experience helping? Where are the boundaries between helping and interfering? Where is our ego in all of this?

- What are the goals of helping? To emphasize self-help and improve coping skills? According to Lawrence Brammer, "The goals of helping have been stated many ways, but generally they reduce to changes in behavior and lifestyle, awareness or insight and understanding, relief from suffering, and changes in thoughts and self-perceptions."[10]

- The art of non-judgment and it's development in the practitioner. The moral and ethical considerations of judging and how to grow beyond it.

- Active listening. What does this oxymoron mean? And how is it performed? What about passive listening?

- What does the reflexognosist do with the information that may be shared or implied?

- What is empathy versus sympathy and when is their use appropriate?

179

- Creating a non-dependency relationship. People want to help one another, and helpers experience deep personal satisfaction through this helping process, but this can create an unhealthy co-dependency situation. Often people wanting to help others actually seek to meet their own unrecognized needs. They may unconsciously set up a co-dependency situation. How can this be avoided?

- What role do individuals play in their own health? Reflexognosists do not heal. Ultimately it is the client who is responsible for his or her health and healing, but we are part of the healing process.

- When do we make a referral to psychologist or other healthcare professional. Where does helping end and playing psychotherapist begin? What can we say without putting ourselves in danger of practicing medicine without a license?

- Self-help approaches. How might individual personalities be helped best? What are some different approaches for the reflexognosist to be aware of?

- The importance of creative self-expression. How can this lead to working through our own challenges and how can it be a tool in helping others work through theirs?

- Self-development of the practitioner. A course on communication can lead to greater self-awareness and development for both the practitioner and, in turn, the client.

- Within the area of communication we can also teach where the boundary of our scope of practice is. Many say reflexognosists are not therapists but can listen like a friend. Friendship is one thing, however, in the role of practitioner, the client is paying you for your services. As a practitioner with your education and credentials you are an authority figure. This puts a different weight on the relationship. You cannot be just a 'friend'.

It is Brammer's contention that, "While there is a need for specialists trained to cope with the complexities of human problems, most human needs can be met by non-specialist helpers."[11] That is, he points out, once they learn a framework in which to view their helping functions. Brammer feels "The two keys to the helping process are the helper as a person and his or her skills."[12]

The client-practitioner relationship lends itself to communications and therefore, it would seem that reflexognosists must include communication skills in their study if the field is going to be acting in a responsible professional manner.

Research

Research which clarifies and validates anecdotal claims and results in new knowledge and ideas is critical to any profession. Only through research will the discovery of the chemical, neurological and other changes taking place with the application of pressure to the legs and feet be uncovered. While outcomes are obvious, the mechanisms by which reflexognosy work, and the link to body cavities will only come through carefully designed research studies. Research will uncover more exciting destinations for us to visit in time to come. Associated with reflexognosy is the Global Reflexognosy Research Institute for Professionals [GRRIP] of Melbourne Australia whose mission is to develop professional foot assessors and investigate the link between structural deviation from normalcy in the feet, body dysfunction, and subsequent health improvement with the use of reflexognosy.

In conjunction with research, there will be calls to discuss reflexognosy from all angles. On-going symposiums will be conducted to allow discussion and debate by leaders in several fields of medical and non-medical teaching to offer their thoughts on the mechanism by which results are achieved.

As a complementary therapy reflexognosy centers on whole health management via the feet and integrates aspects of many other physical therapies, philosophical concepts and technical skills. The journey taken in the curriculum along with other professional considerations leads to an awareness of how dynamic the feet are in the healing process.

[1] Freeman, William H. *Physical Education and Sport in a Changing Society*, 5th Edition. Allyn and Bacon, Needham Heights MA, 1997, pgs. 9-13.
[2] Appelbaum and Lawton, *Ethics and the Professions*, pg. 4.
[3] Ibid pgs. 4-5.
[4] Brookfield, pg. 17.
[5] Ibid. pg. 16.
[6] Appelbaum and Lawton, pg. 8.
[7] Beal, M.C.: "The Subjective Factors of Palpatory Diagnosis", DO 7:91-3, Aug 67.
[8] Beal, Myron C. "Osteopathic Basics", March 1980, Journal of AOA, vol. 79 no. 7.
[9] Brammer. Lawerence. *The Helping Process*, Allyn & Bacon, Boston, 1988, pg. 2
[10] Ibid. pg. 4.
[11] Ibid. pg. viii
[12] Ibid. pg. viii

Reflexognosy Curriculum

1.0 Anatomy and Physiology we are dealing with the physical element.
1.1 Anatomical and Medical terminology
1.2 Gross Anatomy with a lab
1.3 Anatomy of the foot and leg; bony landmarks
1.4 Systems analysis
1.5 Pathology
1.6 Osteopathy principles
1.7 Physiological response to Reflexognosy

2.0 The Role of Feet in Health
2.1 Body cavities concepts
2.2 Biomechanics of leg and foot
2.3 Soft tissue assessment
2.4 Management of the foot including exercises and foot care

3.0 Energy
3.1 Quantum physics
3.2 Subtle energy anatomy encompassing meridians and chakras
3.3 Function and energy

4.0 Tactile Awareness
4.1 From the client's perspective
4.2 From the practitioner's perspective

5.0 Philosophy
5.1 Critical thinking
5.2 The art, science and history of reflexology and development of Reflexognosy
5.3 The nature of illness and healing
5.4 The importance of touch
5.5 The practitioner's role in the healing process

6.0 Legalities in Clinical Practice
6.1 Definition - philosophy
6.2 Scope of practice
6.3 Codes of practice and ethics
6.4 Contraindications
6.5 Informed consent
6.6 Treatment plan

7.0 Business Skills
7.1 Writing a medical report with SOAP Notes
7.2 Making and writing professional referrals
7.3 Case histories for research and development

8.0 Client Assessment
8.1 The five phases of treatment
8.2 Case histories and photographic documentation
8.3 Clinical observational skills
8.4 Podotract analysis
8.5 Post session evaluating of treatment
8.6 Nails and analysis
8.7 Shoe measurement
8.8 Gait analysis
8.9 Case mixing

9.0 Hands-on Techniques - a broader range of application for clinical practice
9.1 Ergonomics for the practitioner
9.2 Positioning and draping
9.3 A variety of Reflexognosy techniques
9.4 Proprioceptive Neuromuscular Facilitiation - PNF
9.5 Joint activation
9.6 Supervised practicum

10.0 Communication Skills
10.1 The art of non-judgment
10.2 Active listening
10.3 Empathy versus sympathy
10.4 Creating a non-dependency relationship
10.5 Relationship of individuals to themselves and the role they play in their own health
10.6 Self-help approaches
10.7 The importance of creative self-expression
10.8 Self-development
10.9 Helping clients through the dying process

11.0 Complementary Therapies
11.1 Essential Oils/Aromatherapy/foot baths
11.2 Basic Nutrition
11.3 Hydrotherapy
11.4 Clinical hypnotherapy
11.5 Massage
11.6 Herbal Medicine

12.0 Research
12.1 Research protocols
12.2 Research projects

Conclusion

"Nothing that is done to the body in the name of therapeutic endeavor should detract from the body's ability to function normally and efficiently."
—Leon Chaitow

The body is self-healing, self-repairing and self-maintaining given the proper environment. Wholistic methods of healing create an atmosphere for the maintenance or the restoration of health based on the recognition of a person being influenced by various factors affecting both their internal and external environments.

All illness is congestive in nature which in turn causes a lack of balance within the body. The goal of reflexognosy is to assist the body in freeing up congestion and encourage balance, not to cure a specific symptom or disease. The reflexognosist will provide the techniques that are conducive to relaxation and assist the body to decongest providing the opportunity to heal.

Reflexognosy is the application of appropriate pressure to the legs and feet by the hands of a trained practitioner to bring about physiological and psychological changes stimulating subtle energies. Portions of quantum physics, biomechanics, podiatry, massage, reflexology, psychology, osteopathy and other modalities are all linked together in reflexognosy to create a wholistic understanding of the body. The effects of palpation are multi-dimensional, effecting the physical and non-physical as different physiological processes come into play. Palpation to the receptors on the feet, coupled with joint activation, produces the range of reactions we see on the physical level. Stimulus travels at enormous speeds and involves very diverse areas of the body. Removal of articular lesions, coupled with hormonal activation, triggering an endocrine response and chakra balancing on the subtle energy level, along with stimulation to the circulatory and lymphatic systems, and all nervous systems, makes reflexognosy a very powerful therapy. Just on the physical level alone at the start, when we palpate we stimulate the nervous system. Then the sympathetic nervous system reacts. By the end of a session the parasympathetic system responds and relaxation occurs. Relaxation of the foot will reverberate up the spinal column and through the autonomic nerve ganglia to the organs and other parts of the body due to the close ties between the central nervous system and the autonomic nervous system. Reflexognosy's ability to assist in decongesting the body via stimulation to the circulatory, lymphatic, and nervous systems directly, and indirectly through the subtle energies housed within the meridians and acupuncture points, assists the vital energy force of the body on several physical and energy planes to balance to the best of its ability.

Any method of wholistic therapy should not have undesirable side effects. Literally, in the hands of the reflexognosist is a most creative, non-invasive, and powerful therapy with few contraindications. Reflexognosists can work with their clients to create an atmosphere in which the body's innate intelligence can choose its own path to healing. Reflexognosy is something that every man, woman, and child may benefit from. In addition, no expensive equipment is needed which makes it affordable to all.

Dr. Simon Wikler had a strong conviction in the feet as the missing link to the health and well being of the individual. Structural deviations from normalcy in the foot will create imbalances which will affect every part of the body, either directly or indirectly. Qualified practitioners around the world are achieving astounding results as the profession grows rapidly. Entering a new millennium, the emerging health care system will integrate manual therapies and reflexognosy will be part of this new model. Research must now commence with the discipline exposed to further academic rigor in order for other health care professionals to have confidence in referring clients to a reflexognosist. Research will also provide a sound and ethical educational foundation upon which to build the discipline.

Therapy on the feet must include an all-round focus—whole health, whole body; a blend of art, science and philosophy. All science, all art, or all philosophy creates an imbalance in itself. The blending of all three is the key, the factor that will create a balanced profession and bring the opportunity for healing to our clients. Reflexognosy is the genesis of a new profession. As the hub of healing, the feet do offer a valuable "Gateway to Health and Healing"

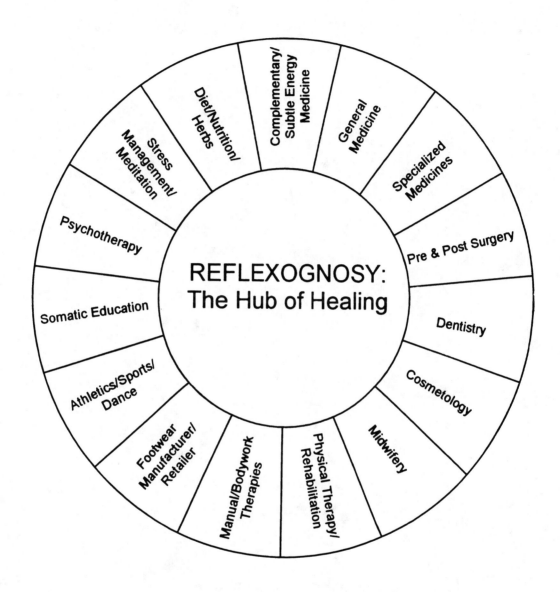

Reflexognosy: an integrative therapy working in a complementary way with all other therapies.

Chart 6

GUIDE TO ILLUSTRATIONS & CHARTS

BIBLIOGRAPHY

Appelbaum, David and Sarah Verone Lawton. *Ethics and the Professions,* Prentice Hall, Englewood Cliffs New Jersey, 1990.

Badawy, Alexander. *The Tomb of Nyhetep-Ptah at Giza and the Tomb of 'Ankhm'ahor at Saqqara,* University of California Press, Berkeley, 1978.

Beal, Myron C. "Osteopathic Basics", *Journal of Americal Osteopathic Association,* Vol.79 No. 7, March 1980. "The Subjective Factors of Palpatory Diagnosis", *DO* 7:91-3, Aug 67.

Becker, Robert O. and Gary Selden. *The Body Electric,* William Morrow and Company, New York, 1985.

Brammer, Lawerence. *The Helping Relationship,* Allyn and Bacon, Boston, 1988.

Brookfield, Stephen D. Developing *Critical Thinkers,* Josey-Bass Publishers, San Francisco, 1987.

Bruyere, Rosalyn L. *Wheels of Light,* Fireside, New York, 1994.

Capra, Fritjof.*The Tao of Physics,* Bantam Books, New York, 1984. *The Turning Point,* Bantam Books, New York, 1983.

Chapman, Frank and Charles Owen. *An Endocrine Interpretation of Chapman's Reflexes,* American Academy of Osteopathy, Newark, OH, 1992.

Chaitow, Leon. *Soft Tissue Manipulation,* Healing Arts Press, Rochester VT, 1988.

Chopra, Deepak. *Quantum Healing,* Bantam Books, New York, 1989.

Clybourne, Harold E. *Journal AOA,* Columbus, OH, February 1931.

Cornelius, Alfons. *Pressure Points, Their Origin and Significance,* Berlin, 1902.

Danaberg, Howard J. *Prevention,* December 1994.

DaVinci, Leonado. *Leonardo On Painting,* edited by Martin Kemp, Yale University Press, New Haven, 1989.

de Saint Exupery, Antoine. *The Little Prince,* Harcourt Brace Jovanovich, Publishers, San Diego, 1971.

Dossey, Larry. *Space, Time & Medicine,* New Science Library, Shambhala, Boston, 1982. *Meaning & Medicine,* 1993.

Evans, Michael & Lain Rodger. *Anthroposophical Medicine,* Thorsons, London, 1992.

Fitzgerald, William H. and Edwin F. Bowers. *Zone Therapy,* Mokelumne Hill CA, Health Research, 1917.

Freeman, William H. *Physical Education and Sports in a Changing Society,* 5th Edition, Ally and Beacon, Needham Heights MA, 1997.

Fromm, Erich. *Psychoanalysis and Religion,* New York, Bantum Books, 1950.

Gerber, Richard. *Vibrational Medicine* Bear & Company, Santa Fe, New Mexico, 1988.

Goldthwait, Brown, Saim and Kuhns. *Body Mechanics in Health and Disease.*

Gris, Henry and William Dick. *The New Soviet Psychic Discoveries,* Prentice-Hall, Englewood Cliffs, New Jersey, 1978.

Grossman, Richard. *The Other Medicines*, Doubleday & Company, Inc. Garden City, New York, 1985.

Ghalioungui, Paul. *Health and Healing in Ancient Egypt*, Cairo, Dar A-Maaref, 1965.

Haeger, Knut. *Illustrated History of Surgery*, Bell Publication, New York, 1988.

Hiss, John Martin. *Functional Foot Disorder*, The Oxford Press, Los Angeles, 1949"Treatment and Care of Feet", lecture at Columbia University, 1938

Ingham, Eunice. *Stories the Feet Can Tell*, Ingham Publishing, St. Petersburg, Florida, USA, 1938. *Stories the Feet Have Told*, Ingham Publishing, St. Petersburg, Florida, USA, 1951. *Zone Therapy It's Application to the Glands and Kindred Ailments*, Rochester NY, 1945

International Council of Reflexologists. "Podiatry & Reflexology: Results of a Study"*1993 Conference Transcript*, Littleton CO, 1993.

Issel, Christine. *Reflexology: Art, Science & History*, New Frontier Publishing, Sacramento, California, 1990.

Karagulla, Shafica and Dora van Gelder Kunz. *The Chakras and the Human Energy Fields*, The Theosophical Publishing House, Wheaton, IL, 1989.

Kastner, Mark. *Alternative Healing*, Halycon Publishing, La Mesa, California, 1993.

King, Francis X. *Rudolf Steiner and Holistic Medicine*, Nicolas-Hays, Inc, York Beach, Maine, 1987.

Kuhn, Thomas. *The Structure of Scientific Revolutions*, University of Chicago Press, Chicago, 1970.

Linden, Millicent. *Stretch for Life*, Information Incorporated, New York, 1968.

Mann, Felix. *Acupuncture, The Ancient Chinese Art of Healing and How it Works Scientifically*, Vintage Book, New York, 1973.

Maxwell, B.C. *Two Feet of Foot Comfort.*

Montague, Ashley. *Touching: The Human Significance of the Skin*, Harper & Row Publishers, New York, 1971.

Naisbitt, John. *Megatrends*, Warner Books, Inc., New York, 1984.

Rick, James A, *Arch Enemies*, Christopher Lawrence Communications, Fargo ND, 1989.

Riley, Joe Shelby. *Conquering Units: or the Mastery of Disease*, 1921

Riley, Joe Shelby and (Mrs.) L. Dow Balliett. *Numerology & Vibration*, Health Research, Mokelumne Hill, CA., 1959.

Robbins, Steven. *Health & Nutrition Letter*, Tufts University, April 1997, Vol. 15, No. 2.

Rogers, Sandra. *Professional Reflexology for Everyone*, Victorian Centre of Reflexology and Training, Victoria, Australia, 1992.
"Reflexology on Trial", *Lifewise: The Australian Journal of Natural Therapies and Allied Health Care*, Vermont, Victoria, Vol. 1 No. 4, December 1993.

Rossi, Laurence and David Cheek. *Mind-Body Therapy*, WW Norton, New York, 1994.

Schaef, Anne Wilson. *Beyond Therapy, Beyond Science*, Harper San Francisco, New York, 1992.

Schultz William. *Shiatsu, Japanese Finger Pressure Therapy*, Bell Publishing Co New York,1976.

Scott, Jane and Ronald Markert. "Relationship Between Critical Thinking Skills and Success in Preclinical Courses". *Academic Medicine* V.69, November 1994.

Stedman, Thomas. *Illustrated Stedman's Medical Dictionary*, Wilkins & Wilkins, Baltimore, c. 1982.

Stevens, Anita and Lucy Freeman. *Your Mind Can Cure*, Hawthorn Books, Inc., New York 1974.

Steiner, Rudolf. *What Can the Art of Healing Learn Through Spiritual Science?*, Mercury Press, Spring Valley NY, 1986.

Triance, Edward. *Osteopathy*, Thorsons Publishing Group, Wellingborough, 1986.

Twentyman, Ralph. *The Science and Art of Healing*, Floris Books, Edinburgh, 1992.

Wells, Samuel R. *New Physiognomy*, Fowler & Wells Co, New York, 1894.

Williams, Tom, *Chinese Medicine*, Element Books, Great Britain, 1995.

Wikler, Simon J. *Walk Don't Run*, Winward Publishing, Inc. Miami, FL, 1980.
"Foot Defects as Possible Etiological Factor in Cancer", *Journal National Association of Chiropodists*, August 1950. "Hypothetical Relationship of Foot Imbalance to Rheumatic Fever", *Journal National Association of Chiropodists*, 1951. *A Guide to Foot Assessment for Reflexologists*, 1990

_____. *Merriam-Webster New Collegiate Dictionary*, Simon & Shuster, New York, 1986.

_____ *The New Webster Encyclopedic Dictionary of the English Language*

_____ *Virtue's Household Physician, Vol. II.* Virtue & Company Limited, London.

INDEX